Published by Maria Paratore

Syracuse, NY

This publication is intended to be a supplement to the advice of your personal physician, nutritionist, or other holistic practitioner. It does not intend to endorse any specific company or product.

For questions or comments please email me at mariaparatore@msn.com

Printed in the United States of America.

Body (and Brain!) REWIRED

Tired Of Being Tired?

Getting your A$$ off the couch and get moving is THE only way to refine your body and your Life!

Introduction

So, you are finally tired of being tired, not happy with how you feel every day, not happy with what you look like in the mirror... Now you are looking for a change...

Now that you are off that couch, I have four questions for you!

My questions for you are: why, what, when, and how?

Why did you pick this book up to begin with, when there are so many to choose from?

What are you looking to accomplish, what are your health goals?

Just as importantly, *when* are you looking to achieve whatever those health goals are?

Finally, *how* important is it to you, and your family, that you reach your health goals?

Why are these questions important to ask yourself? Simply because if you don't know what you want to accomplish, and have a specific time frame to accomplish them by, you'll never figure out how YOU are going get there!

So you want the hard cold truth you say? Well....

Stop Screwing Around!

If you aren't willing to take the time to put to paper the answers to these four simple but focusing questions, then please put this book down, save your money, and go buy another donut, sit back down in that couch and enjoy your life as it is now!

If you haven't put this book down yet, I am thrilled for you!

Let's get started!

To begin with, you are today where you are based on the decisions you have made along your life journey. You are exactly what you think (yes I said think), what you eat, what you have been exposed to, and what type of environment you reside in. Your genetic make-up is a combination of traits passed along from your parents as well as those you yourself have manifested within and around you. While these other contributing factors in your youth (upbringing, environment, parents and their thought processes), have impacted your present state of being, as you grew older you have had the chance to reshape your life. If you've not done so, that's OK! However, the past is in the past and your attitude needs to change right now. Every day you are given the opportunity to start anew! The power to achieve a healthy lifestyle is 100% in your control and that should excite you!

Entitlement. Let's get this straight. You, me, anyone and everyone...We are entitled to NOTHING! I see this attitude in many children and young adults these days that reeks of I should have, I need, and I want, but I won't lift a finger to achieve it. The notion that someone should "cut you some slack" or that you "deserve" something is not only demeaning to your own self –respect, but also sends the message that hard work, dedication, and perseverance mean nothing. The smug, elitist, entitlement attitude will not make you many friends or gain you happiness in life. In regards to your health, nothing is going to happen unless **YOU** start taking responsibility for your own health and well-being. You must humbly *own* who and what you are. So the bragging, bitching, whining, and overall sh&t attitude must be dumped here and now. No one owes you a damn thing, and in fact, you owe it to yourself and your family to be the best you can be in all aspects of your life. Your very best comes from that hard work and dedication to who you are regardless of your hardships, shortcomings, or upbringing. There is no prize for showing up in life, so get used to it, get over it, and let us move forward.

Shortcuts are ONLY for Your Desktop. There are no shortcuts to achieving optimum health and wellness. There are millions of pills, potions, medications, and quick fixes out there you can try. You can read books, magazines, and a variety of other publications that suggest the newest fat loss fads, advertising everything from the soup diet, a protein only diet, to the super fat burner pill.

Go OLD SCHOOL. Think back or ask your parents or grandparents what life was life years and years ago. Allow them to tell you stories of times when people actually had to get up at the wee hours of the morning and put in a full 8-12 hours of hard core physical labor at their job just to put food on the table (some people still do). Students had to walk to school, and then played outdoors when they arrived at home. Homework was done, and families sat at the dinner table together to eat a wholesome dinner. Now, think of what happens in your household. In our present state of affairs, technology, work travel, and our over bearing fears of "over-doing" it are slowly killing us. Kids don't go out and mow the lawn anymore because we are afraid they may "over-heat". Shoveling snow is practically obsolete as we all snow blow or hire a plow service. Children don't play in the neighborhood riding bikes and stick ball because parents are afraid they may get hurt, kidnapped, or have an asthma attack. Video games dominate after school time, and family weekends are devoted to feasting, video games, or in some cases parents forced to work instead of investing in quality physical family bonding time. Sound familiar? Are we just that stressed? Or are we just lazy? The answer may make you think for a moment as to what your lifestyle situation is, and what you are allowing yourself to do and thereby teaching your children. Fortunately and unfortunately, the world has changed. It is a miracle to contact someone across the world in an instant, however, it is also a detriment to our learning and physically functioning abilities that we no longer move or communicate at an optimum level. Why is this important? One of our goals on this earth is to be to be productive citizens and thereby teaching our offspring to do the same. Being productive allows us to maintain a career and lifestyle that we desire with many comforts and luxuries. However, as difficult as it may be to hear, sitting around on our a$$es, playing video games, and eating useless garbage for hours on end is no way to "live". The brain fog, gut rot, and constant sugar craving you reap from such practices highly impedes your ability to be productive and achieve much of anything worthwhile.

Dumping Your OLD HOOD Habits. Think of what you are embarking on as moving to a classier neighborhood. You are becoming "richer" in both knowledge and skill so it's time to "move on up"! Release your old ways of thinking and realize the first step to abandoning such a detrimental lifestyle is to face reality that your body is not designed to work that way! Bluntly put, if you eat sh!t, and drink sh%t, you undoubtedly will look and feel like sh*t! You should therefore not be surprised to discover that you feel "foggy", stressed, fat, overworked, have headaches, joint pain, and in general are a hot mess. What do you think will become of your family if this is the example of yourself you are giving them?

None of the "quick fix" solutions are substitutes for personal growth, hard work, consistent effort, life organization, and structure. Believe it or not we all crave structure. As children in school, we followed a specific plan for the day outlined by the teacher and we stuck to those plans. Morning lessons, physical education class, music or art, lunch, library, snack...Our day was planned. A similar approach with more leniencies was instituted for high school and perhaps college. So as you see, the more we are organized in life, the less stress and chaos we have to deal with. With that said, you are still welcome to run out and purchase all the gimmicks, gadgets, and diet pills you want. You can ask your doctor for bypass surgery referrals or prescription diet pills. You can even go to your local health club and begin a prescribed workout program. However, if you don't "rewire" the way you think, create structure in your life, put in the necessary serious physical effort in, eat healthfully and mindfully, and work on your mental and emotional wellness, chances are that you will be "re-inventing yourself" once again on New Year's Day! Year after frustrating year it will become commonplace to you.

You have seen the New Year's "crowd" at the gym haven't you? Don't they seem to dwindle to only a few once March comes around? They lose, they gain, and they come back the next year for another go-around, right? Well, you can decide to be part of that frustrating routine, or you can be your solution. It's entirely up to you! And it begins with your desire to take ownership of your life and health... That's just the cold, hard truth.

I could mislead you and tell you this is easy. As most of us already know, nothing worthwhile in life is. Whatever your profession or position in life, more than likely you had to strive for, work hard and sometimes long hours, and be an overcomer to achieve those successes. They were not just handed to you. You had to fight for and earn them! So you already inherently know how to achieve success when you put your mind and heart to it.

This journey you are embarking on is no different. Without your vibrant health, those other successes won't mean much. If you have the misfortune of incurring a debilitating lifestyle related disease resulting in your being connected to medical machines in a hospital bed or even at home, what of your career and hobbies will be important then?

If not for yourself, think of your spouse, your children, grandchildren, friends, extended family, coworkers, etc. No one wants to see you ill and suffering. YOU should not want to see yourself ill and suffering. And yes, while some things can't be avoided entirely, so many diseases and conditions CAN! It all begins with changing the way you think, and then relaying the message to your body to take action.

The "easy way" to live would be to sit in front of the flat screen vegetating and stuffing your face with commonly ingested fats, sugars, and useless carbohydrates. While committing to eternal toxicity you could continue to plague your body and brain with useless activities that rob your body and brain of nutrients. If you haven't noticed, it's become increasingly easy and comfortable to be (for lack of a better way to say it)... A lazy slob. It is accepted, embraced, and in some ways encouraged in today's society. We are supposed to love and accept "big as beautiful". There is even so-called research that tries to convince us that being over – weight is healthy. What a crock of crap! Does anyone truly deeply think that carrying around 50 plus pounds of pure fat is actually healthy? The stress on the joints alone is enough to make all that extra "fluff" horribly uncomfortable, not to mention the array of dysfunction that is taking place in your body waiting to attack your major organs. So stop "cutting yourself some slack" and don't feed into the bullsh*t that it's OK to be fat and out of shape. Put simply, it's not, and you damn well know better. Am I advocating you should never relax and share precious tube time with the family? Absolutely not. I am however **not** advocating that you spend 3-4 hours every night eating mindlessly in front of the TV and taking away dinner time at the dinner table with the family. I believe that we should spend some quality family time vegging in front of the TV watching fun family movies or shows together. It's a bonding experience and brings families together for a good laugh. However, as I am sure you have surmised, Americans sit way too often these days. If you complain of lower back pain I am willing to bet you sit in a chair at work most of the day and on your caboose at home a good 2 hours per night. So quit it now and start learning ways to incorporate movement, thereby stimulating your mind and body help to slow the aging process in all of your body systems. Start right now by putting the remote down and limit yourself to 3 hours per week of TV time. Read, walk, play with your kids/pets, stretch, do yoga, go to the gym...SOMETHING! As I am guessing that is the reason you picked up and started reading this book...To change!

Yes, this all may be harsh, and matter of factly, but who else is going to kick you in the caboose and tell you honestly which direction you should take? You can't rely on the biases of media, or those so-called "research studies" sponsored by "Independent Medical Firms" steering you towards the latest 'do-nothing, eat everything, and lose weight fast' product (only to discover those "Firms" are owned by the product's manufacturer!). You can't rely on the slick advertising of the food giants telling you about how healthy this new cereal or that new weight loss drink, or that new prepackaged healthy all natural food, or 'nutritional' breakfast bar is. Whole grains? 100% natural?...I'll let you in on a secret. Most of these "claims" are 100% bullsh%t! So much of what is considered "healthy" out there is genetically modified, laden with fillers, unidentifiable chemicals, hormones, trans fats, sugar, and crap your body can't and won't use to nourish itself.

And I'm sure you've seen the late night (why are you still awake then) infomercials about this new "machine" that will tone you up, or trim your fat, or build muscle in '15 minutes a day", as you see the picture perfect models demonstrate how effective the product is! Do you really think that those models got those bodies by using that product only? So what is one to do? How do we sift through the nonsense? Good question...Here is the answer: Stop believing everything you see on TV. If it looks too good to be true, it probably is. If you can't read, spell, or understand ingredients in the food you are buying, DON'T buy it! PERIOD!

You may think processing the truth, putting together and implementing a plan into action is very time consuming and challenging if not impossible. Yet, we all have careers, children, and demands at home, family, hobbies and causes we believe in that are integral to the make-up of who we are as a person. Many of us work 8-10 or more hours a day, and then it's on to taking the kids to practice, a game, or school event, not to mention our own events. We feel we need time to unwind, to take care of our homes and families, and because of this we more than likely let ourselves go. *Sound familiar?*

While many use these as motivation to get our a$$es moving, MANY others are using them as excuses for not devoting the time and effort to change the way they live to improve their lives and lifestyle. If you are still reading, you probably have been in the latter group and just believe there has to be more to life than that. Now is the time to change the way you think and fall into the former group! Remember this, the choice is always yours!

There is a better more fulfilling way to live, but only IF you are willing to change the way you think and what you do! Think of how much better of a mother, father, grandparent, sibling, spouse, or friend you can be to others when you radiate positivity and a healthy glow? Think of that day you proudly walk your daughter down the aisle, or wait for what seems like forever at the hospital to meet your first grandchild!

Think of the times you've returned from a warm sunny vacation. Were you refreshed, well rested? Feeling relaxed, invigorated, healthy, happy, and positive about your life? I'll bet you were! Now transform those feelings into your everyday living by treating yourself to a healthy lifestyle.

Does devoting 4-5 days a week for 45 minutes to 1 hour per day of fat burning, muscle strengthening, and stretching, coupled with a healthful nutrient rich diet and some stress management sound like a challenge? It will be at first, until you become aware of the benefits for you and your family.

What this really comes down to is your **PRIORITIES** in life! In reality, it's never a time problem, and it's not really a knowledge problem; it's a *priority* problem! It's human nature that people will find the time to do the things they WANT to do, yet be unable to find the time for things that aren't high priority to them! It's just that simple. Finding that time whether it's the early morning hours, later in the evening, at lunch, or even in the few free moments throughout the day, are small contributions to you in exchange for vibrant energy, health, and well-being well into your old age. Why cozy up to the idea that you should just be resigned to living life day to day, and give in to the "I'm too old, I already have done that, and there is no hope for me" mentality. That line of thinking will totally and completely manifest a less than ideal sense of well-being. Why accept the following: orthopedic issues from lack of muscle strength, joint stress due to excessive weight gain, an aching body where everything hurts, high cholesterol, hypertension, diabetes, and cancer, just to name a few!

Do you think you can live a happy and vigorous life eating junk food and taking more and more prescribed and over-the-counter medications, with the lack of energy to enjoy quality time with your partner, children, grandchildren, and other friends and family? Will you have a good quality of life while suffering with hormonal imbalances or those that are unresponsive, and everything from thyroid dysfunction to lack of libido that may plague you as you search for answers, quick fixes, and band-Aid approaches to these issues?

Now maybe I'm sounding catastrophic, but that is not my intent! I'm not trying to scare you into a better life and a healthier lifestyle. Will any or all of these horrible health conditions really affect you? Maybe, maybe not. There are so many contributing factors that are individual in nature such as genetics, environment, and what you have done with your life up to this point to name a few! Are you a gambler? Playing Russian roulette with your healthy, happy existence seems hardly a wise option.

Instead, are you ready and willing to get off your caboose, leave your baggage and drama at the door, and start actually living rather than existing?

Every day you are blessed with the opportunity for a fresh new start to the rest of your life! You can go out and healthfully live that beautiful life of yours and have a vibrant fulfilling existence, or you can let yourself go and live uncomfortably. The best part is...the choice is yours. You are not fated to lifestyle related diseases. You may have a few genetic or orthopedic limitations, but we all do. If you are truly not limited by any severe health implications, then there is nothing to hold you back. If you have limits, learn to live around them and how to accommodate them without causing further damage. Hopefully at this point you are beginning to see why you are in this position in life and how you can begin to change. So let's move on to who the hell I am and why I am so passionate about your life as well as my own.

So why should you listen to me? Because it's all about you!

Allow me tell you a little bit about me, and then you can make your own decision whether who I am, what I have done, and what I'm about is relatable to you and what you are seeking. After all, life is about relationships, and relationships are built upon trust. By telling you my story, I hope you will begin to trust that I truly have your best interests at heart.

Firstly, there are millions of fitness "gurus" out there who have constructed credible publications that have helped many people succeed. Now I don't know that I would call myself a "guru", nor has anything tragic or special happened to me that catapulted me into this life long quest. As a child, I always strove to be active and athletic. It was something I needed to work very diligently at, as it didn't come naturally to me. I was never extremely proficient in any one sport. Yet I discovered fitness at a very young age, waking up early to perform my morning dose of home or gym workouts before school. I was a soccer player and had the huge legs to prove it. I strove to become leaner and fit as a young high school student emulating the lean athletes in magazines. I became an advocate of health and fitness incorporating a variety of activities into my life. In high school, I decided my desire was to work in the field of physical activity, and went on to attend SUNY Cortland majoring in Physical Education with a focus in Exercise Physiology. I then continued at SUNY Cortland where I completed my Master's Degree in Health Education. Career wise, I began working in a fitness facility, while also in corporate wellness. I had the opportunity to work closely with physical therapists and many other holistic health professionals. Today, I am 39 years old and am in the best shape of my life. I have taught physical education for more than 12 years. I have competed in, and won 3 bodybuilding competitions. I am an avid runner, track coach, group fitness trainer, personal trainer, sports therapist, and Reiki Master. There is nothing uniquely special about what I do or the knowledge I have acquired throughout my life. I have simply followed my passion! I am humbled that many people have benefited from my having been given the chance to serve them and to share this knowledge with them. I am honored that these people trusted me and my commitment to improving their lives through my practice.

My purpose here is to share what I have learned over the years with you as well. It's about giving you the tools to achieve YOUR goals. It's not about me or what I have accomplished. Without those who could benefit from using this helpful tool, my efforts would mean absolutely nothing. I would like to thank everyone and anyone who reads this publication, as I feel honored to have this opportunity to share all of this wonderful information with you. Much of this information I have acquired over the years comes from the personal experiences of me and those that I have worked with. I will do my best to direct you to the sources in which I have obtained all of this information, however, my trial and error over the years will be to your benefit.

I also must clarify that I am not a doctor and am in no way giving medical advice. Nor am I asking you to follow what I am sharing with you in place of what your doctor is telling you. I am however asking that you consider doing as I have done, fully educating yourself about how the body works, and what alternatives are available to you. I encourage you to seek therapies and remedies that are not neatly packaged in a pharmaceutical pill. I ask you to be open minded and refrain from thinking there is some "magic pill" or "quick fix" approach to health and life. Be intellectually honest with yourself. There is no drug, surgery, diet pill, non-effort protocol, no eat whatever the heck you feel like diet that will give you the results you seek. I only ask you to consider what I and the many I have helped have done, and embrace the reality of "hard work", consistent effort, and implementing this approach to finally get to the fitness, fat, and level of health you desire.

The suggestions in this book are compiled from real life experiences and interactions with holistic professionals who have made a huge difference in my life while on my journey for health and wellness. I hope the information in this book serves as a valuable reference for your life long journey to wellness. With the utmost sincerity, I offer my experiences, efforts, and knowledge with the hope that you find this as beneficial in your life as I have in mine. Again, thank you for allowing me to share.

Work and play your heart out... and never ever stop.

Chapter 1: Right to the Point...We are So Going There!

Here, I am going to list in great detail some life lessons I have learned that have enabled me to live my life happily, healthfully, and with the best physical results I could achieve. There are many topics of interest and all are important in combination with each other. I have tried to explain each point in as much detail as I believe will allow you to use the information provided without being overwhelmed. There will be enough information to make good decisions, but as previously mentioned, I recommend educating yourself more about each topic. Keep in mind this is about helping you change your lifestyle, and there is no possible way to include all the available information for each topic here. As this is merely a starting point, think of this as a self- paced course to a better life. This is a lifelong quest, not a stroll in the park! It is useless to start and stop something just to return to your former existence. So this is not "a diet". You are not going to partake in this lifestyle for a few weeks and be done with a new body and life without ever having to put in another stitch of effort. Again, your body just doesn't work that way.

I hope you find that what's presented is as valuable as I have. Please understand this, I will not provide you with garbage information or so called quick fixes. I will not tell you it's going to be soooo easy. There are no trophies for just showing up (nor should there ever be, but that's another story). Your trophy will be what you will be able to give to your family and those important to you because you are living a health positive life!

Along this exciting journey that is your life, even when we think we are working our hardest (and we very well may be), things will not always be perfect. You will have to roll with both the good and bad times. Winning and losing in the variety of situations that appear in our lives teaches us valuable lessons, builds our character, and makes our accomplishments that much more meaningful. Having challenges, and overcoming them is what makes the achievement that much sweeter in the end. Your body and mind are more capable of overcoming stresses and challenges than you may realize. Once you come to terms with the realization that your body is a rather unique machine, the faster you will be able to set yourself up for success. So, if you are up for the challenge, I'm up to guiding you as close to success as I can without being right next to you.

So back to the questions you should have been thinking over....

WHY? The MOST important thing, without question, is you must have a powerful enough reason WHY you need this change! Once you have found your why, then it becomes about priorities. It becomes a priority issue, never a time, cost, pain, appearance, age, history, eating, or learning issue!

What is YOUR reason, your WHY? Write it down, put it on the fridge, put it on the bathroom mirror, put it in your car, or carry it in your wallet. Keep your WHY visible so you never lose sight of it! This is important to help keep your focus.

Is your WHY to be there for your family and children and set a healthy example for them? Maybe your goal it to be there to walk your daughter down the aisle? Or is it to be there to play with your grandchildren, your family legacy? How about being an athletic into your 70's and beyond? To look good and feel better while searching for that person you want to share the rest of your life with? Maybe to stay healthy as you move up the corporate ladder and all the added stress, time, and work to get you there? Everyone's WHY is going to be different, but achieving it needs to be your highest priority.

If your WHY isn't big enough, if it does not eat at your core, your soul, your inner being until it hurts, then nothing else will matter. You'll put up the good fight for a while, but you'll eventually make 'legitimate' excuses why to miss a day or two or more. The day or two will turn into a few days, then a week, and before you know it you won't remember the last time you did something. You'll lose your momentum and quit, going back to how you currently are (or worse), probably more defeated and frustrated than before you started. The worst part then will be that you'll convince yourself that it's not that bad as you are.

PMA.   Going hand in hand with having a powerful WHY, you MUST change your way of thinking to a **Positive Mental Attitude**! You are going nowhere fast if you think negatively. You will over-think and worry yourself fat and helpless, not to mention the stress you are putting on your heart and digestive system. Read about and put into practice ways to approach and conquer negativity in your life. Publications such as "The Law of Attraction" and "You Can Heal Your Life" by Louise Hay are good starting points. Look up Dr. Wayne Dyer since he has a huge selection of life changing reading material. There are many more, but these are some of my personal favorites. You are what you think you are, and what you project to others. If you call yourself fat, and think you amount to nothing... Guess what? That is exactly what you will be manifesting in your life. Abundance is a natural state in our life. The well- known saying: If you think you can, you're right! If you think you can't, you're right! We reap what we sow and create a deep seeded reality in our minds. Our negative and limited thinking brings us to scarcity and misery. Now, getting on the "positivity bandwagon" is not some hocus pocus bull crap that is going to immediately get you to that svelte and healthy physique without actually working towards it. Achievement of any kind is a two-fold process. Number 1, believe in yourself, number 2, get out there are start living it. So at this very moment, get rid of the beliefs that paralyze your positivity and you are halfway there. Get your thought process on a positive track, become enthusiastic about your life, and you will begin seeing many successes in all areas of your life.

Believe me, I know this is the most difficult thing for someone to accomplish. There are many positive things already in your life, but the negativity of your thoughts clouds your vision to the point of not being able to see or recognize the many great things you have going for you and around you!

It's relatively easy to change physical part of you. It's the deep-seeded mental and emotional beliefs we hold consciously and unconsciously that have an enormous impact on our lives. Start educating yourself on how to tackle those beliefs which limit your success. By doing so, you will begin to create the life that you want for yourself within your body, mind, and spirit. The positivity you radiate will spill over into other areas of your life.

For example, try thinking of what I call: "Little Victories!"

When you made the decision to improve your health, get a celery and carrot cup instead of a candy bar, walk around the block instead of driving, or taking the stairs instead of the elevator, the first time you go to the Gym, Fitness Center, or break out your own equipment and begin working it (no matter how good or bad it goes), getting a book or looking online for healthy meals and snacks you can make at home, going back and working out a second day, deciding to have some grilled or baked chicken and veggies instead of that five topping large pizza, drinking water instead of soda (diet included!), having a hard-boiled egg instead of that deliciously sweet Danish in the morning, all little victories! How about when you suddenly notice that you have to tighten your belt to the next hole? As you can already see, you already have double-digit victories on your journey to a better and healthier LIFE! How exciting is that?

Finally, do you know anyone who just has it all together? Do they seem to have a "flow" about them that just exudes confidence and positivity? Guess what? You can do that as well! Start by thinking positively and eliminating all those negative thinking patterns. You will be amazed at the results.

Remember, you are what you think you are!

BE REAL. This goes along with thinking positively. Regardless of *who* you are, regardless of your undying will power for success, we all break down. Give yourself what I call a "recovery period". This "recovery period" doesn't include being a candy ass and downing a half gallon of ice cream.

Here, I am asking you to take a time out for yourself. Sit down, take 10 deep breaths. As you do that, imagine breathing in white light (which is healing) and exhaling black smoke (all the negativity). If you need more than 10 breaths take them. Lie down if you need to. Diffuse the insanity, which will help you to "recover" in many situations. This can be done at your desk, in the shower, bathroom, waiting in line at the store.... You get the idea. I am asking you to resist the super defeated "negativity mode" when the kids miss the bus and the dog soils the carpet. Another "recovery period" idea is to give yourself 5 minutes. Sit down, stretch, meditate, listen to your favorite song, or watch a funny clip online. Take your mind away and remember sh*t happens and it happens to ALL of us. You can't fix everything in one day. You have to look at what needs to change for you, and then make a plan in order of importance and ease of ability to change. Some things take more time and effort than others. Small changes, tackling one problem or health concern at a time yields greater success in the long run. Small successes (Little Victories) build our confidence and turn into large milestones over time.

GET STARTED!   For the love of the universe.... Do Not Wait! Procrastination kills the spirit and momentum of your decision to change! All the New Year's hype is so overplayed. "New Year, New You"...BALONEY! Start right now! RIGHT NOW...THIS MINUTE! Don't fall into the "I'll start Monday crap. Start NOW! Even if it only one small change to get things started! What's stopping you? What's the worst thing that could happen? We are all busy. It's about prioritizing your decisions. You can make the conscious decision to start right now. You can start by taking a walk at lunch or skipping the fatty latte this morning. You have the power of choice. Finding one solution leads to one better choice. One good choice leads to a second, and a third, and you see where we are going with this. (Remember the 'Little Victories' I mentioned earlier.) You're on a roll.

I GOT THIS! Don't depend on others for your success, nor blame them for your failure. Your failure or SUCCESS rests solely with you. Yes, it's great to have a buddy or honey to workout with. It's vital to have someone be accountable with. It's also beneficial to have a personal trainer, group fitness instructor, or nutritionist to motivate and educate you. However, do not use them as your crutch. When that go-to person is not around, moves away, or falls off the wagon, what are you going to do then? Are you going to quit? Will you still get out of bed at 5am, even in the cold, snow, or rainy weather, and make it to the gym anyway? Or instead, will you sleep in and later kick yourself time and time again in frustration and anger? Do not depend solely on someone else for your success. Take control and commit to yourself (once and for all) that you are going to do this for you, and nothing will stand in your way.

STRESS AND COPING. We touched on this previously, and I asked you to use a "recover period" when the sh*t hits the fan. Now, I ask you to learn your most intense stressors and develop effective coping skills to work through them without resorting to self-sabotage such as devouring a box of cookies when the going gets tough, or lying in bed sulking for hours. That is the easy way out as we know, and remember, we discussed this may not always be easy. I have learned over the course of my life that in the midst of crisis, it is always best to keep in mind that somewhere someone else has it worse than me. There are soldiers fighting wars, people living in horrible conditions, children starving, and people who have lost limbs or one of their senses such as their eyesight or hearing. There are people with cancer, or other terminal diseases that still hold onto hope and positivity each and every day. They live their lives happy to be alive and so should you! So if you really think about it your crap really isn't that bad. Crazy and horrible road blocks pop up on us all the time. An aging parent falls ill. The hot water tank fails, the car has issues, the kids have problems in school, and your boss is driving you crazy. Even things like divorce, bankruptcy, accidents, job loss, all of it, most of us have gone through something. Yeah, yeah, it's supposed to make you stronger so they say… we know. Maybe it's a lesson and there is a silver lining you need to look for. Thinking along the lines of "there is a reason for everything" will encourage you to look for this silver lining. Situations or people that leave us open doors for new and better situations to arrive. Think of it as cleaning you're your closet and opening your windows letting in fresh air. Does that sound easy? It may not be in reality, BUT that's the first step in the right direction. You have to sit yourself down to re-evaluate and know there is light at the end of that dark tunnel. Frame of mind is everything. How can you distress? Will excessive eating, sleeping, smoking, drugs, or alcohol take away the problem? Be honest, you know they won't!

 Here are a few suggestions to consider in times of crisis. Try journaling, talking to a friend or family member, go for a jog, do sprints, take a boxing or yoga class, engage in spiritual activity, hug your pet, meditate. Remember no one's life is perfect (you see that in the tabloids). Embrace what is happening and focus on a plan to take care of you in times of great stress. Find your "Happy Place", go there when needed, and thank yourself for handling the situation with a more levelheaded approach.

LEARN ABOUT YOUR BODY. Research other medical and medicinal philosophies. Modern medicine has often left our bodies in shambles after polluting it with toxic medications that in many cases only relieve the symptoms and not the root cause of the condition. When researching, be sure to take into account where the research is coming from. Who is funding it? Medical companies? A product manufacturer? It is very easy to be misled in a product or practice being very good or very bad based on who is writing the article or funding the research. There are groups of people out there who seek to keep us dumb, fat, and medicated, so please research carefully. Seek out unbiased research that clearly identifies the true benefits and disadvantages to using a specific medication. Ingest medications only when ABSOLUTELY necessary or your life depends on it! I am not in any way again stating you SHOULD abandon medicine and freely do as you wish ingesting herbs and tinctures and mindlessly hoping for the best. I am repeating that because I want to make it clear that certain medications may be necessary for people to live or overcome a specific illness. For example, if I incur a staph infection I am not going to solely rely on homeopathic remedies to fight the infection, I am going to take my antibiotics and nurture myself with probiotics and food to fight the infection and keep my digestive system in check. However, I am not going to run to the doctor every time I get a sniffle and walk out with five prescriptions. See the difference? If my lower back is stiff or sore, I may stretch, do yoga, lower back exercises, or take a hot bath with Epsom salts. My first go to should not be pain meds. That's the concept we need to embrace. Our bodies will thank us for it now and for years to come.

The "Root" of the Problem

Oddly enough, it is worthwhile to mention that if you look carefully at credible research you will realize that many diseases start in the spine and the colon. Did you know that the majority of your immune capabilities are in your gut? So if you are riddled with stress, smoking, bad eating habits, soda drinking, or ingesting an excess of stimulants and other medications (just to name a few) you are setting yourself up for disease and disaster. At first, you may feel stressed or tired. Tired becomes exhausted and cranky. Tired and cranky may lead to a cold or the flu. And chronic "mini-illness" begins piling up into one big bang! The horrible and possible result is high cholesterol, high blood pressure, ulcers, clogged arteries, or even a heart attack or cancer. What you eat and drink has a huge impact on your health if you haven't had that hit home by now. The medications, both prescription and over the counter have an impact on your body's organ systems to function appropriately. I can't stress enough that we as culture feed our need for that quick fix approach and seem to run to the doctor or drug store for pills at the slightest discomfort instead of addressing the real problem. Lack of sleep, vitamin and mineral deficiencies, stress, poor eating habits, chemicals we ingest, the environment, all of these things play a role in our body function, and almost all of them we have control over. Our body's immune system, when functioning efficiently can destroy most incoming pathogens and bad bacteria. Our bodies naturally make painkilling substances and antibodies that fight disease. Think of all the diseases that you know of and where they originate in the body. Why do you think it's recommended that you get a colonoscopy by age 50? How many people do you know that have back issues such as bulging, herniated or degenerative disc disease? Think about when you are constipated. That is not an appetizing thought, but really we have all been there, think about what is going on in your body when you are constipated. Toxins are just filling your body with no pathway to exit. That's what's happening. Therefore, it is essential to take care of your colon. There are a variety of ways to cleanse the colon and protect the spine and you will find you are healthier, more energetic, and in a lot less pain by doing so.

Let's look at some other topics by group. I have grouped them by Food, Physical, and other types of therapies

LIVE IT....Today

Juice!   Get a juicer, the more sophisticated it is, the better the quality of the juice. However, if money is tight, a less expensive one will do. Get one and *use* it. See recipes for a quick healthy simple juice at the back of this book. I highly recommend the Vitamix or Ninja, however they run around $200-$400. What are you going to put in your juicer? Easy! Start with a combination of fresh fruits and veggies (preferably organic) so that you are starting to ingest more vitamins and minerals every single day. Drink your juice fresh every morning. This will help you to start boosting your immune system and energizing your body. Most juicers come with a booklet to get you started on what combinations of fruits and veggies to put in your juicer. Great combinations such as kale and pineapples, or apples spinach and a banana may sound strange at first, however juiced together taste divine. You can use berries, mangos, carrots, beets, the list goes on. Here is where you can be creative as well and make up your own combinations, or look online for some new and interesting ways to juice.

Read the Labels Please!   Read the labels on everything and anything you buy at the grocery store and get to know what you are putting in your body. Most restaurants have nutrition information available now as well on their menus. As I cringe saying this, if you must visit a fast food establishment, get to know where and what is good to put in your body from such places or you will find yourself smothered in grease and chemicals. Keep in mind many processed foods become addictive especially in the form of sugars and starch we find in breads, drinks, canned products, cereals, and the list goes on and on! You will need to prepare by mindfully grocery shopping and pre-preparing meals so you are sure to incorporate more organic GMO free products in your diet, the less ingredients the better. Just as an example of what NOT to do… Blue #4 and yellow #5 are not naturally occurring substances; therefore, you shouldn't consume them. Look for things you don't recognize in the label ingredients and chose products that are not brimming with chemicals. All of those "sugar-free, low-fat, low carb" products are GARBAGE! Most of them are designed to have either more chemicals or if its low fat it has more sugar if it's low sugar it has too much fat (and not the healthy fat)…you get the idea. Keep in mind that not all products listed "organic" truly are. Learn about GMO's (genetically modified organic) and how to avoid them. Truly organic foods will have far more of the good stuff you want, without the bad stuff you don't! (Remember about educating yourself?)

To expand on that "sugar-free" thought….

Stop eating fake sugar.   You know the stuff I am referring to! It's the junk with zero calories or sugar alcohol that wreaks havoc on your digestion and prompts you to crave more sugar. These are chemicals altered to be low in calories but just as unhealthy as bleached sugar. In moderation, use raw cane sugar, raw natural honey, or stevia, they are natural, safe, and won't prompt you into a sugar addiction. Just as another FYI, many diseases and conditions feed off of the sugar we ingest. Cut the sugar and you will notice you crave it less and are dramatically decreasing your chances of suffering from a variety of different diseases and conditions.

Avoid the High FRUCTOSE Corn Syrup   Look for and try to avoid this crap called high fructose corn syrup. Yes, there are claims that it is "like any other sugar", but just as fake sugar, it's processed, it promotes sugar cravings and overeating. It possesses nothing you need in your body, and breaks down into many toxins you don't want. Although natural forms of sugar are best, keep in mind any type of sugar ingested in excess from food you eat will dramatically increase blood glucose levels (blood sugar). In turn, your body's insulin levels will begin to rise. Insulin is produced in the body to lower your glucose and help store what is not needed. However, constant elevated blood glucose levels are symptoms of diabetes, heart disease, stroke, high blood pressure, cancer and obesity. So that's another of many reasons to kick that crap to the curb!

Regulate your electrolytes.   What are they? They are potassium, sodium, magnesium, calcium, and chloride most importantly. Your kidneys play a vital role in regulating these vital substances. Nothing will zap your energy faster than the electrolyte imbalance. How do you fix that? Start with water. Drink enough water. We actually should be consuming up to a gallon a day. We rarely get there. It is essential to replace electrolytes after vigorous exercise. You don't have to use a sugary drink to do that. Don't be fooled by Sports drinks! Check the labels, and you'll find many of them have as much or more sugar in them as a soda! Start with drinking water before, during, and after exercise. Unless you are competing in a lengthy endurance competition, water is the best choice you can make! Be sure you replace what you have lost with a good (think healthy) balanced meal as well. Your metabolism is at its highest after vigorous exercise. Since you are most depleted at this time, this is also the time to have your largest meal of the day.

Dump the excessive starch.   No, I am not asking you to go "carb free" or start starving yourself on an unrealistic "diet". We all know that "Diets" don't work! So let's forget the "diet", and start adopting healthful blood sugar regulating nutrition. Unfortunately, many of us get confused as to what it is, and what or how we should be eating to lose body fat. So many people think eating oatmeal for breakfast, rice or bread with lunch, and pasta for dinner is healthy. Well yes, it is healthier than eating fried food or creamy, fatty sauces. However, to lose body fat, too many starchy carbs interfere with blood sugar regulation leaving you hungry and tired. Hence, the idea of decreasing the amount of starchy carbs by eating them only with one meal of the day can be extremely effective. Additionally, it's even more effective to replace some of those starchy carbs with fibrous carbohydrates (green veggies) and increasing the healthy fats and proteins (Avocados and Salmon for example).

Dump the alcohol!   Yup, I know you should INDULGE once in a while! Yes, you should! HOWEVER, twice a week 3 glasses of wine, is just way too much. Alcohol slows down your metabolism because it is a depressant. That's a fact. Yes, a glass of red wine now and again is good for you (organic is best). Just as organic dark chocolate is good for you in moderation (80%+ cacao is the best). The bad news is that you can have too much of a good thing. Having one or two glasses of wine per week (not every day) is harmless. If you can refrain from downing a brick of cheese and box of crackers to go with it...by all means enjoy! View it as a special treat such as on a special occasion or a Friday night date. The rest of the time, drink some water with lemon or herbal tea. That is much better for you, and a lot less expensive!

Bump up the healthy oils and fats.   There is a hideous misconception out there that eating fat will make you fat. This is simply not true. Of course eating trans fats, and man-made forms of chemical junk that you see listed as ingredients on food label, or deep fried food does not constitute eating healthy fats. Bump up your HDL (good cholesterol) and keep yourself full (by not munching on useless sugar and carbs all day) by increasing your healthy fats. A teaspoon of almond, cashew, or natural peanut butter is a great treat with your yogurt, in your protein shake, or on your occasional organic multi-grain toast. Avocados, Extra Virgin Coconut Oil, Ghee, and pure, organic extra virgin olive oil have proven to be excellent sources of healthy fat. Other examples are walnut oil, avocado oil, and fish oils such as that from wild salmon. There are many more I have left out, but these are the main sources that I have used with great success.

Eat More Healthy Protein. Experiment with different sources of healthy protein. Experiment with taste and effect. Are you vegetarian or vegan? No problem! There are so many choices out there why not try them all! You can find plenty of vegan options in the department of protein and milk. You name it, it's out there. My little secret to a yummy smoothie is pumpkin. Yes organic canned pumpkin in a chocolate or vanilla flavored shake is just smooth and creamy. You can choose to use whatever healthy options you desire. We will talk more about what those options are later on. Just remember use natural sweeteners if needed, not the "fake sugar".

Apple Cider Vinegar? Oh yes.. Take apple cider vinegar. Sound absolutely disgusting I know, however, you will be amazed at some of the things it can do for you. Take 2 shot glasses per day of organic apple cider vinegar with "Mother" (the silt like solids) mixed with your water or tea. Add another shot of organic lemon juice for a double detoxifying effect. It is important that you use the most natural kind. In addition to it contributing to your weight management, it will also aid in digestion and ward off any stomach illnesses by killing off any nasty bacteria in your gut. (Remember that most of your immune system lives in your gut!) For those of you who have sinus conditions, it's helpful with those as well.

Eat More Vegetables. Mom always told you to eat your veggies. And she was right! In addition to juicing, eating more fresh organic vegetables is filling, satisfying, and duh...healthy. I specify organic because it should be evident by now that ingesting fewer chemicals and pesticides will undoubtedly improve your health and longevity. This is pretty much common sense. During the nicer weather, consider creating your own garden as it can be very fulfilling as well as budget friendly. You may also seek out local farms for produce delivery to your home, or visit your local farmers market to find fresh veggies with less carcinogenic (cancer causing) chemicals that pollute your body. You should have at least five servings of vegetables every day. When trying to lose body fat, it is more effective to utilize more of the cruciferous veggies as they have more fiber (so they are more filling) less calories, (so you can eat more) and pack a punch of healthy antioxidants. Some examples are kale, broccoli, cauliflower, arugula, and cabbage. Although not on that list, I believe spinach to be a super food because of its versatility and nutritional content. It is also very convenient to grab a bunch for salads, smoothies, or to steam or sauté lightly. All of these are great cancer fighters as well. Experiment to discover your favorite way to prepare any of these (and more) and don't be afraid to try something new!

Take vitamins with green foods. In addition to eating more green foods, I personally recommend taking organic multi-vitamins with green foods. Why you ask if you are eating a variety of fruits and veggies? Good question. Remember this: even if your diet is perfect, if you are the model of health and wellness in every form... you may not be getting exactly everything you need from food every single day. It may be impossible for you to eat as much as you need to repair and replenish your body. And if you did, there is no guarantee that the food you are eating, even if grown in your own back yard has 100% of the nutrients you need. Soil and environmental conditions as well as food transport can degrade food nutrients, so why not have an insurance policy? You may say "but if I don't use what's in the vitamin I will excrete it". Yes, in theory we usually excrete what we don't need. If you are thinking of it as wasting money, here is my plea to you. If I were you I would rather pay a few bucks for my insurance policy every month (just like on my car) and have peace of mind knowing I'm getting the proper nutrients and fighting disease, rather than play Russian roulette with my health. So you ask... is a vitamin going to prevent disease? No. However, again, building a bullet-proof immune system will allow you to more effectively fight off any "bad stuff" you encounter. In turn, you may escape from many common illnesses (colds, flu, etc.) with very little or no effect on your well – being. Now, just to clarify, I am not a doctor and will never tell you to stop taking medication, nor would I want you to take something that will interfere with any medication you **must** take. However, I urge you to consult with a holistic doctor who will truly advise you how to manage medicine with supplemental nutrition. Green food supplements along with actual green foods themselves and antioxidants lower the body's free radical and acidity levels. This can aid in healing as well as will help avoid or reduce the incidence of disease.

Probiotics: Most if not all of us at some point in our lives have had to take anti-biotics to cure and infection or post-surgery to prevent one. Although a truly beneficial substance for that purpose, they are overused almost just as much if not equally as much as pain killers and muscle relaxers. Educating yourself on the use of any medication is something all of us should do..period! Anti-biotics do not kill viruses, therefore, if you have a cold you should not be taking them as colds are viruses. Medications as well as the ingestion of crap food and environmental toxins mess up the health of your gut. If you think you are doing your tum-tum any good by scarfing down that processed garbage they call yogurt at the grocery store, think again. Most commercial dairy products as we have previously discussed, are all pasteurized. While that may sound good for killing off the "bad" bacteria, it also kills of the good stuff as well. And what are you left with? Creamy crap basically. Just like pasteurized milk but in a more solid fermented form. Other issues associated with many "probiotic" yogurts is that they are either not potent enough, made of artificial ingredients, or not really effective in promoting gut health. Artificial junk pretty much leads to the other two reasons for the most part. To be put simply, if you enjoy your yogurt, look for the organic versions that have "LIVE" probiotics. They may be more expensive, but at least you are getting yogurt that is better for you minus the nasty hormones and fake ingredients. There is research that has indicated that it is nearly impossible to keep live strains of necessary "good bacteria" alive in our yogurt even if it is organic, so we may not be getting as much as we need. If in doubt, and you feel the need to ingest additional probiotics, you can try organic kefir, which is a more liquid form of yogurt said to have more probiotics, or other fermented foods including miso soup, tempeh, or Kombucha tea. There are organic drinks specifically designed to include probiotics that are free of sugar and other nasty junk that are quite tasty and refreshing. How do you know if you need more probiotics? We all could use them, however if you have just taken a round of anti-biotics or had a stomach flu, I would suggest using them to restore a healthy digestive balance. Apple cider vinegar here again, is also something to consider restoring intestinal balance and help to knock off any bad critters in your tummy.

PHYSICAL ACTIVITY- Those Weights Are Not Going to Move By Themselves!

How to do it properly...effectively and efficiently.   Learn proper form in your physical craft: biking, running, weight lifting, yoga poses, etc. and don't ever compromise on doing it correctly.

Understand and put into practice exercises and workouts that are challenging to your heart and muscles (walking aimlessly on a treadmill is not going to help your bottom line). Examples I like are: Boot camp style classes, interval based biking classes, boxing/kickboxing, high Intensity Interval training, circuit weight training, plyometric, calisthenics, and body weight exercises.

Do yoga.   Try the "Hot House" style yoga. It's challenging, you stretch, strengthen, and get your Zen on. The room for this activity is very warm and inviting so it's an excellent choice for winter workouts. I enjoy this activity during the dead of winter when it's too cold to do outdoor activities. Mixing up your workouts and keeping your body "guessing" allows it to become stronger, more balanced, and more fit in a variety of ways.

Cardio as opposed to (yawn..) cardio! Stop pretending to do cardio for hours. Tons of 'cardio' will not help you lose fat. In fact, too much will make you so hungry you will want to knock off a burger joint on the way home from the gym. Slow moving, boring, zero challenge, and no variety will not work either. Unless you are training for a specific event, you should not be doing more than ½-1 hour of cardio per day. Better yet, I recommend using "High Intensity Interval Training" instead. This form of cardio is far superior to an hour on the treadmill or elliptical, and can be completed in 20-25 minutes! What is an example of HIIT you ask? One is doing 4-6 30-second sprints with a couple minutes between sprints. Additionally, you will need to challenge yourself for 30 minutes to an hour. Walking or running hills, stairs, jumping rope, boxing, boot-camp class, spinning...the list is endless. Pick something you can tolerate to like or love and let's get this started! One day a week of a moderate pace cardio exercise such as the elliptical trainer or bike is fine. Just remember to mix it up and use your weapons wisely. You have four...Frequency, intensity, time, and type. Keep your body guessing and keep it challenged!

To simplify and intensify your workouts, consider using an app on your smartphone (if you have one). There are a variety of training apps that will time your workout, give you mileage, paces, exercises, music, short, long, cardio based, or strength based workouts. Some apps mix the two. Others even let you chose your own music to set the workout. And many of these apps take into consideration you may not have a huge space or equipment to use. Given all these choices and conveniences at your fingertips there are even less excuses or bull crap reasons why you can't work out.

Don't Sit On Your Caboose! Stop sitting on the bench at the gym and resting. Why? Unless you are a power lifter, let's keep the calories burning shall we? Do some core abdominal work, or lunges in between each set or exercise. How about some jumping jacks or mountain climbers to keep that fat burning up in between your bench presses? One way to really maximize your efforts is to make a "check-list" workout. I do this to ensure I do everything on the list and give myself a time frame in which to complete it. For example, I may have a list of 15-20 exercises to complete in 45 minutes. This may include 50 jumping jacks, 25 squats, 10 minutes of jogging, etc. Be creative! Make the most of your time and efforts by continuing to work. Keep in mind that even activities like jumping rope, high knees, squat jumps, and burpees are all effective in burning that fat. Who cares what people in the gym think? You can bet they will be following your lead when they see how great you are looking. *Interesting tidbit of information I learned years ago:* One pound of muscle burns 35-75 calories per day. One pound of fat burns 9 calories per day...period.

Additionally, many recent credible studies are showing how just sitting for hours at a time at work is actually bad for your health! You can research the data from places such as the MAYO Clinic and the British Medical Journal to get the results of numerous studies of how the way your body processes your blood sugar, triglycerides, and cholesterol while standing and moving as opposed to sitting. Check out the research and look for ways to reduce your daily sedentary time (from a physical activity perspective) this as well. You'll be surprised how much better you'll feel in the long run!

Alternative Therapies

Alternative Thinking. Downing a bunch of pills that cause more side effects than good effects is no way to live and you know it. And what's worse, the drug companies know it. Watch those commercials and look for the side effects of all these drugs you see advertised on TV. And by the way, since when do we have to advertise drugs? So we can go ask our doctor to prescribe them to us?? Really? Now back to the side effects. I am not sure about you, but headaches, nausea, and anal leakage do not sound like something I would like to experience. How about you? I'm guessing those are not your idea of a good time either, yet if you have seen pharmaceutical commercials, you are familiar with these types of statements that are conveniently snuck in at the end. And I would be horribly surprised if you hadn't seen a drug commercial as they are on at least ten times per one hour program. Although these and a variety of other side effects exist, people still run to their doctor for their prescriptions thinking this is the ONLY way to survive. If you think all pharmaceuticals are safe and "effective" at "curing" your ailment, take a moment to think about cigarettes. Can you think of anything healthy about cigarettes? It is a known fact they are carcinogenic, which means they can cause cancer, so why are they still widely available for purchase? I bet you can guess why and the answer has dollar signs written all over it! With that said, it is imperative that you yourself start right now advocating for your OWN health. Do not be bullied into taking crap you don't need or that will cause you more harm than good. So how can you do that without putting yourself at risk? Research, investigate, and try alternative remedies and therapies to deal with minor health issues. Try not to run to the doctor every time you have a sniffle, ache, pain, or can't sleep. As you have surmised, the overuse of medicine runs rampant in the United States. Yes of course sometimes you very well need to take a pharmaceutical if it is the absolute only way to feel or get better. The goal is to try to avoid regular overuse of these substances causes dependency and disruptions in the digestive system not to mention a whole plethora of potential life-long complications that maybe irreversible.

Think of how we overuse anti-biotics again and how it kills off the good as well as the bad bacteria in your digestive system. The potential result is candida overgrowth (a fungus that lives in your mouth and intestines) in your digestive system which can lead to bloating, yeast infections, and constant sugar and carbohydrate cravings. This is just one minor example of how the overuse of medications can lead to additional health problems. So before running to the doctor and begging for a miracle pill, research some natural home remedies that may help you. Try massage or chiropractic for aches and pains or even an Epsom salt bath at the very least. Everything from physical therapy to acupuncture, acupressure, Reiki, Yoga, Meditation, Deep breathing techniques, Visualization, and hundreds of other practices and techniques that I have failed to mention can improve everything from your state of mind to your state of body without the side effects of medication.

Get a massage. Tension and tightness can interfere with body functions internally and externally. You may favor one side or your body or another causing muscle imbalances, and/or other orthopedic issues that drag you down. Let someone pamper you once a month. Massage is also good for lymph drainage and sinus issues.

Consider colon hydrotherapy. Yes, sounds disgusting! Don't think toxins don't get backed up in the colon and cause a number of different problems throughout the body. Though it may sound gross, a good cleaning can leave you feeling "less toxic" and help promote a healthy colon and fat loss. If medically safe for you, find a good hydro-colon therapist to explain this further to you and help you along on your journey to a healthy colon. If this is something that is not for you, consider (if medically safe) an organic colon cleansing product that will eliminate toxins in a similar fashion from your system leaving you feeling less bloated and more energized. Most general practitioners are unfamiliar with this procedure and may advise against it. However, like everything else recommended here I suggest doing your own research and determine if having this procedure makes sense for you.

You have that juicer so why not try...

Juice Cleansing? Consider a fresh juice cleanse for 3-10 day depending on your tolerance to eliminate toxicity from your body and help repair digestion. Juice cleansing takes a lot of will power and mental strength to achieve. It does however provide a sense of clarity both physically and mentally. After about three days, cravings and brain fog cease, digestion issues begin to dissipate, and you feel as though your body is "regenerating" itself. This is not for everyone, so if you have any doubts about your tolerance for such activity, or if you take medication, please again consult a holistic doctor who can determine the appropriateness of this type of cleanse and who will monitor your efforts.

With that said... yes juicing is wonderful, but do not use that crap in a bottle or carton! Make your own from fresh ingredients (with no preservatives). There are many great recipes you can find with a little bit of effort to suit your taste.

Yes, I just said drink juice, BUT, as an overall "rule" it is best to limit drinking your calories. Here I am referring to the fatty lattes, juices in excess (especially ones that are not fresh, and check the sugar and extra ingredients), milk, creamers, soda, beverages with fake sugar, and especially alcohol are all something that should be used in extreme moderation like a special occasion. Save the milk for your protein shakes if you use them and do fresh juices once a day or during a detox. The rest just add empty calories to your daily intake without much help to fill you. Drink water with lemon (for cleansing purposes) and herbal teas.

Some MORE thoughts regarding milk... While growing up we all had milk for cereal and to drink with meals being told it was good and healthy for us. Just like yogurt almost all of the 'normal' cow milk we drink is homogenized and filled with the hormones that were administered to the cow the milk came from. And guess what? You are now ingesting all of those hormones and chemicals as well! If you think the "processing" of milk sterilizes it and makes it safe it doesn't. And there are so many mustache milk ads that try to convince you of the many health benefits of milk. Bullsh$t! It is comparable to drinking sewage as many of the nutrients that naturally occur in cow milk are removed during homogenization. Between that and the hormones and anti-biotics given to these poor animals, you are basically left with mucous and garbage that is not very healthy. If you are worried about calcium, eat some spinach. If you need your milk "fix", experiment! Though slightly more expensive, it is worth considering other options such as flax milk, almond milk, cashew milk, and even hemp milk. There are plenty more I am not mentioning here. Beware of added sugar in the flavored nut and seed milks as you don't need to add more sugar to your diet. Many of these milk alternatives have a creamy delicious taste and keep more of the nutrients without the fat of regular, even skim milk.

Find a Reiki practitioner. You do not have to believe in Reiki to benefit from its healing properties. Reiki is a Japanese form of energy healing. The practitioner places their hands on the energy centers of your body for periods of time to transfer energy which feels like heat. Some practitioners do not actually make contact with the body and this is determined by their previous teachings and client preferences. It can however have a profound healing effect on the body and has been used for centuries to rebalance and allow the person to heal themselves.

Take a Detox Bath. Try a bath with Epsom salt (2 cups), baking soda (1 box), and authentic tea tree oil (10 drops). Sounds interesting doesn't it? Well it is actually a really good idea. The Epsom salt is soothing to the muscles and joints. Research as shown that magnesium and sulfate when absorbed through the skin may have a great deal of benefit to the body by reducing inflammation, flushing toxins, improving the function of nerves and muscles, and reducing the pain of migraine headaches. Tea tree oil is a substance that is anti-fungal and antibacterial. It is a natural substance that can be used to treat small scrapes and other wounds to cleaning your home. A few drops in a bath are great for killing bacteria. According to a holistic nutritionist that I visit, baking soda is used for eliminating radiation from the body.

Speaking of detoxifying the body, have you ever heard of .....

Infrared Sauna Therapy. This alternative therapy has been the craze lately with infrared sauna therapy studios popping up just as tanning salons used to. What is all the madness about getting sweaty in a wooden little hut? Although not a new concept, it has been recognized that infrared rays have the ability to penetrate the body on a deep enough level that not only promotes healing, and allows for detoxification of all the body's systems. Infrared therapy has shown to have the ability to boost our immune systems, help relieve muscle soreness, improve arthritis, and aid in weight loss. There is a variety of research out there that attests to the benefits of using an infrared sauna. They don't "feel" as hot and unbearable as a traditional sauna, and deliver relaxation as well as a healthy dose of infrared therapy. As with any other type of alternative therapy, you should do your research and/or ask a holistic practitioner if this would be of benefit to you. Keep in mind individuals who must take certain medications may have some contraindications regarding the use of infrared or any saunas for that matter and must be sure to mind that recommendation. Additionally, it is imperative to drink plenty of water during and after your session to ensure you do not dehydrate. To find some quick and easy information on the subject, this site proved to be helpful to me:

http://www.globalhealingcenter.com/natural-health/health-benefits-of-far-infrared-therapy.   I myself have visited an infrared sauna studio and can attest to the fact that my muscle soreness has significantly decreased, I have slept sounder, and felt very invigorated after my session. Home based infrared saunas are also available for those who would like to reap the continuous benefits in the comfort of your own home. There is no concrete documentation that clearly states how often and for how many minutes one should use infrared sauna therapy. Individual needs, preferences, and recommendations from a holistic therapist are all ways to determine frequency, intensity, and time in regards to use. I have used a sauna up to times per week for 45 minutes per session with progressive elevation in temperature up to 145 degrees. As the time decreases, the temperature decreases. This is a program set within the sauna itself that can be customized to one's tolerance.

Holistic Health Care, the best there is. Find a holistic health care professional you trust. It is important to take the time to educate yourself about this, remembering again this is part of your lifelong journey. How do you know you can trust them? Start by asking them questions regarding their ethics and treatment procedures. If they are pushing pills and painkillers on you for minor ailments, or they are bashing vitamins and supplements, walk (no RUN) away!

Are you sick of walking into the doctor's office for a minor ailment and walking out with five prescriptions? Did the doctor actually sit and talk with you regarding your condition or did you give most of your information to the nurse and visit with the doctor for all of three minutes? This is extremely important. Yes, doctors are busy people. Nurses are a vital part of their practice as they are there to collect information and check your vital signs. Nurses are an integral part of the practice and having known many, they are amazing people who do more than they are ever given credit for. However, it is essential to build a rapport with the doctor who is making the diagnosis and recommendations regarding your well-being.

For me, I really want to know that person and how they operate. Do they have a comforting "bed-side manner"? If it is too much for them to spend some time building a relationship with their patients, then it's best that you find someone who will do that for you. There are plenty of general practitioners out there who maintain a holistic viewpoint and will be open, honest, and up front with your regarding medicine. Make sure you are asking questions!

Also, I suggest writing your questions down before you visit your doctor. This way you are less likely to forget to ask something important to you! And for heaven's sake, do NOT think that you'll ask him/her next time. If it is something that bothers you do not be embarrassed to ask and talk about it. If you don't have that comfort level, to discuss anything with your doctor, then you probably need to find another doctor that you are that comfortable with!

I have an interesting story that goes along with why I believe this is important. Right before I attended college I went to my primary care physician for a physical. I was asked a few questions, the nurse assessed my heart rate, blood pressure, etc., and that was it. I left the office with not one, not two, but three, yes, three prescriptions. All for things I didn't complain about at all. I received two medical prescriptions for allergy medication, and one for a birth control pill. All of which was unnecessary, as I didn't need any of those medications at the time. It was because of this incident that I realized I needed to be an advocate for my own health. I started to do my own research in conjunction with my studies at SUNY Cortland. During that research, I learned about and found many holistic professionals such as nutritionists, massage therapists, hydro colon therapists, Reiki Masters, and the list goes on. I discovered that these individuals were proactive, not reactive when it came to maintaining optimum health.

See a Chiropractor. I would recommend seeing a chiropractor for an alignment if possible. A little Snao-Crackle-and Pop can go a long way! As you know from biology class that your nervous system runs through your backbone and out to your limbs and torso. This is important to understand that while all your movements, your heart and lung functions, your digestion, your ability to do anything and everything physically starts in your brain, but it's the nervous system that sends the signals from your brain throughout your body that makes things happen. Electrical signals to your heart to keep pumping, your diaphragm to keep breathing, even to your muscles that control your fingers to type on your computer. Over time through lifting, carrying, running, sitting, falls, accidents and just general moving around, your bones get out of alignment. In some cases they get so far out of alignment that you'll hear of pinched nerves, and for some just feeling weaker or general discomfort. A good chiropractor will analyze you through posture, x-rays, range of motion assessments, and such and will let you know how your alignment is, and make some recommendations before actually doing anything to you. In some cases, just a monthly or quarterly adjustment may be all that's necessary. For others they may need multiple adjustments to get aligned properly and improve how their nervous systems run their body. Once you are back in good alignment, you'll be surprised how much better you'll feel overall.

Get your hormones in check. Surprisingly, estrogen, progesterone, testosterone, and your thyroid hormones (among others) all have a significant impact on your body composition. Although it can be difficult to assess at what amount some hormone levels should be at in your body, there is usually a range that is "normal". When you have a physical, request a profile of your hormone levels, and ask what range they should be in (if there is one). If there is an imbalance, ask what your options are in regards to improvement.

Another condition worth mentioning is something called "adrenal fatigue". This happens when your adrenal glands (located on top of your kidneys) basically get "burned out" leaving you tired, foggy, irritable, and unable to have the "drive" you normally would. Adrenal fatigue can be serious and is caused mainly by a significant amount of stress. It is imperative that you check to see if you are at risk for any of the above hormone deficiencies and learn how to rebalance them naturally if possible. One immediate way to help your wacked out hormones is to dump that nasty sugar habit. It always comes back to sugar doesn't it? Yes! Get rid of sugar, and consult a holistic professional such as a nutritionist, doctor, or homeopathic professional to discover how to improve your hormone function.

Get Your Home in check. Clutter? Disorganization? Crap everywhere? This entire cluster of sorts invades your physical and mental ability to focus and find what you need when you need it. Don't use it? Get rid of it! Organize your crap, keep your home clean and tidy, and have a place for everything. File important papers and personal information. Clean out closets of unused debris and donate it all to charity or have a garage sale. Believe it or not, this can be very liberating and allow you to stress less when looking for more important items.

No Drama Here! Don't become, or stop acting like a drama queen/king! Are you one of those people who always have drama and trauma? Do little things make you fall into a pool of negativity? Do you live for gossiping about everything from your family situations to officemates? Well stop being a hot mess! No one likes to deal with negative Nancy, Bill, Bob, or whoever you are. Learn patience, learn to control your emotions, and learn how to be happy in productive when the crap hits the fan. One good tool to channel your emotions of course is exercise. Another is meditation. For some it may be yoga. Talk it out; leave your gossip and baggage at the door. I definitely believe that negative talk including negative self –talk not only impedes our ability to bring the positive to our lives but it also clutters our mind with useless crap when we could be focusing on the parts of life that really matter...Friends, family, loved ones...OURSELVES! Don't worry and focus on what others are doing. If you do, you should sit yourself down and figure out why you are so interested in what others are thinking rather than focusing on YOU! If you find yourself falling into a trap like this, sit down and write out 5 things that you are thankful for. Use gratitude as your weapon against negativity. Write it, say it, and really mean it! Be happy you are alive and have the ability to read this book and understand how to use it, be happy for your family, your pets, your friends and loved ones, your career...and even the lessons you have learned that have led you to the right here and now. Be grateful and thankful, and do this each and every day. You will be surprised at how liberating it is. Another idea would be to write or say daily affirmations like: "I am happy, joyous and abundant in all areas of my life", or "Everything is right in my world right now, I am exactly where I am supposed to be". Try it, you will be surprised.

Hate ain't great!   To drive that last point home, here is another good piece of advice. Don't be a hater! Stop judging, ridiculing, poking fun at, being jealous, nasty, or any other hateful attitude you exude. And forgive! Forgive yourself, your family, friends, "frenemies", or anyone else you have wronged or have wronged you intentionally or unintentionally. It is freeing to let go of all that has built inside you. Do this deep within your soul and you will see the weight drop off mentally as well as physically. If you judge others and hold hatred and "unforgiveness", you will hold the weight on your body as well as your mind as they are so very connected. Forgive yourself, forgive others. Trust me on this. Stress hormones and all will haunt you in mind, body, and soul.

Chapter 2

NO! Mediocre (aka being "Average") is NOT Ok

Getting Your A$$ Away From Excuses…

For many of us overworked/underpaid type 'A' personalities out there, we have organization down to the last minute of our day and have everything planned for the next week. Even as we have become natural "micromanagers" of our time, we still often encounter obstacles that really interfere with our ability to properly take care of ourselves. Of the many road blocks we can discuss here, the most common denominator among many people are those little bundles of joy we call CHILDREN! As wonderful and rewarding as they are, well let's face it, they can run any high-energy person ragged! One is a handful, two or more and you are seriously impeding your time and efforts to be fit and healthy. Well let's cut through that nonsense…

In most families both adults are working with very few stay at home moms or dads anymore. Two incomes are almost always essential to live comfortably, or for many to get by at all. Mom and dad may be working 40 plus hours a week, cooking, cleaning, laundry, getting little Joey to practice on time, grocery shopping, and play dates. Single parents are saints for being able to juggle their lives and those of their children minus a spouse. By Friday, if you actually have a "normal" work week, everyone is exhausted. Now throw in a few games, weekend yard work, perhaps shoveling in the winter months, or a home project, and you can bet you are beat to a pulp come Sunday night. In just sharing these few facts, we can start to realize our obstacles. Now we must learn how to work around them.

So how do we do that?

Glad you asked. Let's start by imploring two very important principles...

#1. Despite an overwhelming array of responsibilities, we must train ourselves to say the word "NO". Saying "NO" is ok! Remember how we discussed earlier the importance of having priorities! There needs to be a list somewhere ingrained in your consciousness, even better if written down, that tells you what NEEDS to be done and whose NEEDS must be met. Remember that YOUR health needs to be your priority. Without your health you will struggle taking care of all the other priorities including properly taking care of and setting the example for your children! So if there is no impending need... it's ok to just say no, or not at this time. You could spend your entire life at PTO meetings, neighborhood gatherings, jewelry and candle parties, company golf outings, or other events that you would rather skip anyway.

Immediate family/friends events and traumas, of course are a must. No one would ever tell you to shut out someone close to you or not allow them to depend on you. That is not only selfish, but very bad karma. (You get what you give, don't forget that). However for some, it is just as easy to just feel bad for not making the garden club meeting so that you can bring your famous chocolate chip cookies. You need to have a life too. In my profession, it is vital to be there for those who need me. I have spent countless hours trying to rearrange my life and schedule to fit everyone in and make everyone happy. It never happens. At the end of the day someone is not getting exactly what they want. I have to just step back and realize I am one person, and if deep down I believe it will all work out...it usually does! Don't go feeling guilty either. I will bet my house that no one you know works as hard as you and pleases everyone. It just can't happen. Politely say no and move on. You will be surprised that most of the time everyone will understand and have been in the same situation. There will be other times you can lend a helping hand. Those important to you and who care for you will understand and work with you. Those who demand your time without consideration are only looking out for their own agenda.

#2. To complement principle #1, learn to put yourself first as much as humanly possible. Yes children need their parents. A sick parent or a spouse who may have just had surgery needs family for moral and emotional support. That doesn't mean your life goes to complete hell for that period of time. The loss of family members or even your family pet can be utterly devastating. To this day I miss my boxer named Zero. She was a loving gentle soul whom I still cry about occasionally. When I lost her, I felt an emptiness that couldn't be fulfilled with any amount of food or comfort from others. We have all lost pets, grandparents, aunts, uncles, friends, or even our parents or children. In all cases, it can feel physically and emotionally debilitating. We must realize they are in a better place and would want us to go on healthy and happy. At any time you are experiencing any type of loss keep in mind you are only as good to those you love and support as you are to yourself. There is nothing that can take away the pain of loss except time and more importantly how you spend that time. Staying fit and healthy physically and mentally will help you cope with your loss and allow you to be a solid support for others. A good workout could also be a good distraction and help with your emotions. Even in less extreme circumstances, you can't possibly be patient, tolerant, compassionate, or even fun as a spouse, parent, child, etc. if you are an emotional train wreck.

Putting these two principles into practice will be a process and will take time. The more you can utilize these principles the more time you will find for yourself. Now, what to do with that time....

Stop Wasting Your Time; Maximize Your Efficient and Effective Use of It!

For many people who are looking to make the most of the little time they have, the first change they should institute is to make time for exercise. Some people choose to get up a half to an hour earlier a few days per week just so they can spend some time focusing on the workout and not everything else. Yes, it is true your rest is very important and skimping on sleep will have a negative impact on your ability to concentrate, your mood, and eventually your metabolism over time. So you will have to be smart about this.

Some tips for getting a peaceful rest and a productive tomorrow. Know what time you plan to get to bed, and half an hour before then put down the phone and resist the urge to look at your social media sites or any games you play online. Read a book or meditate to help get you in a mental state to rest. As far as television goes, limit it to 1-3 hours per week. The garbage on TV will just pollute your mind most of the time anyway, not to mention, you have more important things that you could be doing with that time. Think about it. Do you really want to live your life through the lives of the fictional characters on TV anyway? I know this will be much easier said than done, so take little steps at a time. If you watch 4-5 hours a night, cut back by picking one or 2 shows and use that time to prepare for the next day or read. You'll find out that many of the shows you watch only because they're on! If you must, you can always TiVo or Hulu to watch them on the weekend, so you still gain that time during the week.

Secondly, get the kids situated and to bed. If you have no kids, this is bonus time to do things to better your life. If you have a dog, taking a short stroll and getting some fresh air will be good for the both of you. You may even chose to learn something new, read; perhaps this is the time to get your workout in...

Thirdly, if you haven't done so already, get your lunch ready for tomorrow, as well as getting your workout clothes and work clothes ready to go. This takes some of the fussing and rushing away from the morning when you are still trying to wake yourself up and be ready for the day. If you've prepped in advance, your morning stress level goes away! Just to ensure I don't miss workout opportunities, I always leave a fully "loaded" gym bag in the car. I fill it with sneakers, socks, shorts, yoga pants, shirts, sweatshirt, underwear, shower accessories, and even a running, jacket, gloves, and hat. I keep in there year around just in case! It serves a two-fold purpose. Number one, heaven forbid you ever are stranded somewhere with your vehicle broken down and no cell service. You may need some of these items! Secondly, if I forget my workout items, I already have some... NO EXCUSE to skip that workout!

Lastly, get to bed. The more time you can get in sleep mode before midnight the better. If you work odd shifts or rotating shifts, you can still do all of the above and get yourself to bed at a time that allows you to rest for 6-8 hours. If you work the more 9-5 shift, ten O'clock should be the latest your buns are in bed unless the sky is falling, or for some dire emergency your work/child schedule doesn't allow that. Watching the last episode of your favorite gossip show doesn't count and it just may lead you to eating something naughty right before bed. I will confess, I am the biggest violator of this rule yet I always feel better when I get to bed by 10 pm. I am slowly breaking myself of my night owl patterns. Staying up too late not only leads to overeating, but also hitting the snooze button, abandoning the morning workout, and feeling exhausted all day. You may relate to this, I even retain water all over my body when I don't sleep enough. So resting appropriately is the key to waking up refreshed especially if you are an early morning exerciser. Some people can truly only find time in the morning to work out and de-stress so don't pass this time up or feel like its death to get up in the morning. Some people may even have to get up at 4:30 am just to have 45 minutes to an hour of sweat time before the rest of the family is up begging for breakfast. You have to do what works for you and remember, no one ever said it would be easy.

 Does this mean you can never sleep in again? No, it shouldn't mean that at all actually. What is should mean is that you are budgeting an allotment of time for yourself to be healthy and fit. It's time for you and you alone; however it doesn't need to be every day of the week either. Getting a workout in 2-3 days during the week, then possibly finding some time for you 1-2 days over the weekend to be active for an hour should be plenty for most people unless you are training for something specific. This of course may vary depending on the number and severity of "obstacles" that come up that may attempt to throw you off your schedule. Making a point to establishing a routine will prove to be helpful regardless of circumstances. This is why having your priorities specifically identified is so important! Again, your priorities should be in alignment with achieving your "Why"! Give yourself a solid month on this plan and I am betting you will find you feel better, are more energized, and will feel like "ah..It's working"!

 Early morning workouts can be a challenge to get used to, but when you are finished you have a sense of accomplishment knowing it's DONE for the day and you have the rest of the day to truly focus on other important things in your life. This sense of accomplishment, plus a fit and healthy body, is the inspiration for many thriving groups of runners, workout partners, and group fitness classes. You can find like people to push you and be accountable to just by soliciting a friend, someone you work with, a neighbor, sibling, or other family member to join you. You don't even have to join a gym (though for some it's better, for others the gym becomes a social club)! Find a great DVD, an APP on your phone, or a nice versatile piece of exercise equipment to use at home. If all else fails, check out the website www.meetup.com, you can find TONS of groups of people in your area that literally meet up to do activities such as mountain biking, hiking, running, or even mountain climbing. There are even health/weight loss groups, holistic and homeopathic wellness groups, and many other non-physical activity groups. Having people like yourself all in the same proverbial boat can prove to be fun, cool, and meet your fitness needs within your schedule. Even better, it's a great way to add new people and other interests into your life!

If you really would like to get creative, consider starting some group exercise at work! If you have a flexible or long enough lunch hour, instead of everyone stuffing their face for an hour, why not walk for 45 min and then eat lunch before returning to your desk? Some workplaces have worksite wellness programs, wellness centers, and flexible working times so that you can come to work later after working out but stay later to work, or come in early for work, skip a break and leave early so you could go workout. In my own school district, I started an after school workout class that was originally designed to be a sports conditioning class for athletic teams. In designing the class, I created group workouts that integrated sports conditioning with aerobic and strength training. This combination allowed me to participate with my students, giving us all a great workout. The next thing I knew, it was catching on to the rest of the teaching staff. I ended up having staff district wide come to participate in this after school class. We had a blast! The kids enjoyed seeing their role models sweat and work hard beside of them! So as you can see, you may need to be creative and explore other avenues to get the right fit. Most people find success taking one of the above venues. We are not looking for a time that is convenient, because let's face it, there is NO real convenient time; if that's what you are waiting for let me assure you, it will never happen. What you are looking for are ways to make the best use of your precious time. You can always make more money and more friends, but once you have used your time, you can never get it back! And living a healthy lifestyle adds value not only to your life, but to your ability to help others as well. You may even add many years to your life by changing to a healthier lifestyle!

Chapter 3:

The Eating Quandary

Well here we are again talking about food. Now let's get a bit more specific. I don't know about you, but I am not down with high cholesterol, high blood pressure, heart disease, diabetes, or cancer (just to name a few). Busy or not, people always find this one to be the most challenging aspects of beginning to change their lives. To make matters worse, no one knows what the hell to eat or not eat anymore, in which case we want to throw our hands in the air and commit to a life of ingesting hot dogs. As such, we can never have enough discussion on nutrition. I can tell you this, catching a bite here and there in between feeding the kids and laundry does not constitute a balanced meal. What exactly is a balanced meal these days? We have had the food guide pyramid, and then we switched to "My Plate" as a guideline for nutrient intake. "Everyone" is telling us not to eat carbs or wheat, but dairy is killing us with the hormones, and the fake sugar, and high fructose corn syrup, basically all the issues we have covered earlier, here they are again.

 When you do finally make the decision to eat something, and you have found foods that you will actually eat, now you have to try to find some time to sit down and eat. Right! Good luck you may say! When kids are rushing off to school, everyone wanting something different to eat, you are trying to cook, clean up and get yourself to work...it's an interesting, challenging, and sometimes a downright frustrating daily juggle. Getting back once again to your priorities, and remembering that it's okay to say "No". What this should really be about is the value of having meals everyone will eat, and ideally at least a couple times a week where the whole family sits down and eats together with no distractions. No phones, no TV, no radio... just some quality family time together!

If you're single, there's dinner with your family or close friends. Because we have become such a 'mobile' society, this will probably be awkward at first, but in the long run, it's all about family and the people you love.

Instead of mindlessly stuffing your face and sprinting for the door, what you need is an exit plan. By this I mean plan so you can get yourself and everyone else fed appropriately, healthfully, and on course for proper digestion. Here you can utilize that low-tech/high-tech blender that's been collecting dust on the counter (or more likely tucked away in the back under the counter). Not everyone has time for egg whites, sprouted grain toast, oatmeal, or gluten free pancakes. They sound delicious and are wonderful for you; however, in the real world it won't happen until the weekend...maybe.

Many of us don't have time for a five-course breakfast so we have to be creative! Think home-made smoothies! We discussed smoothies earlier, now for the nitty-gritty of what you should add to your smoothie! For optimum health and taste, add your choice of protein powder, milk, and water, with optional fruit, yogurt, or nut butter, maybe a little ice and blend. Thirty seconds later you have breakfast! I have even tossed in a quarter cup of oatmeal occasionally so that I have some healthy carbs and I feel full longer. This is something you can even make the night before while you are preparing lunches. There are so many ways to make a healthy and delicious smoothie, just think of all the ingredients you can add to maximize your health benefits while providing a feeling of fullness. Proteins include whey, pea, hemp, rice, and the list goes on. For liquid, in addition to water you can try different tasty milks such as soy, almond, flax, quinoa, coconut...I am not even close to naming them all. Other delicious additions could be flax or chia seeds, spirulina, and plain organic yogurt or a kefir, which is a more of a liquid type of yogurt that is almost free of lactose. For healthy fats as well as fullness, adding a tablespoon of raw almond, peanut, cashew, or sun butter is a great idea or certain flavored smoothies.

As far as the rest of your days' meals, you have probably figured out by now planning what you are going to put in your mouth ahead of time allows you to monitor your food intake. Blindly, mindlessly eating leaves you overeating, leaving out nutrients, and sets you up to be hungry again within a short period of time. High protein, low sugar snacks minus the nasty fake sugar high fructose corn syrup, white flour and white sugar, are the key to balancing your blood sugar and staving off cravings. Hummus and veggies, an apple and two tablespoons of raw nut butter, a serving of organic vegan cheese and fruit or veggies, even an organic, low sugar energy/protein bar (remember you can make those too) will all be quick and easy. Switch things up with main meals. For carbs consider organic grains such as quinoa, millet, or lentils instead of pasta and white rice. Try including some wild salmon or bison if you eat animal products. Tofu or organic ground turkey can be used for making burgers instead of ground beef. A hearty soup in the crock pot loaded with veggies for those cold winter days, vegetarian or turkey chili, veggie loaded salads, fruit salads, nuts, avocados, legumes, butternut squash, and sweet potatoes are all good ways to add variety to your meals. All delicious, nutritious, and can be prepared in so many different ways you may be overwhelmed for a while trying them all. Start planning your grocery shopping list according to meals for the week, stick to the list, and save appropriately for the good organic stuff if possible.

The message here is stop wasting your money on crap you don't need and put it toward the things you should be putting into your body. Plan your meals ahead of time by shopping with a list at the grocery store and stick to the damn list! Ideally, you can work toward planning the entire week's meals ahead of time and if possible even prepare them ahead of time to heat up for your dinner. Don't worry; you'll get better at this over time. Take the time to learn what's best for you and your family. Remember, no one became an expert overnight! Casseroles are a perfect example of a meal that can be prepared ahead of time and just baked for 20-30 minutes before dinner. All the prep work is finished and the making of the mess in the kitchen is minimalized. Think of organic rice pasta or maybe quinoa or corn pasta with some grilled chicken and veggies and a light homemade marinara sauce. Mix all the cooked ingredients, spread evenly in a baking pan and cover with tin foil. When you are ready to warm it up, put in in the oven with some fresh mozzarella if you do dairy (organic, non-gmo, hormorne/anti-biotic free is best) and bake until the casserole is hot and the cheese is melted. A one dish meal the whole family will enjoy. The crock pot is king when it comes to the concept of cooking ahead. Hearty soups, meat dishes, veggies, sauces, chili, even entire meals can be cooked in the crock pot on low all day and be hot and ready in time for dinner.

Another treat to prepare for the whole family is a batch of healthy granola bars. Make them on a Sunday night, get the whole family involved! Rolled oats, organic raw honey, raw nuts and seeds, raw nut butter, and some extra virgin coconut oil cooked together on the stove and spread nicely onto a baking sheet to chill produces some seriously awesome snacks. These little slices of heaven can be simple, tasty, and healthy. Now everyone including you is happy and the whole family can help out. When you get into a routine of preparing ahead you will start to realize how convenient life will be even when stuff happens. Even if the dog just crapped on the floor, the kids are running around the house screaming, and the basement floods, you've got this! You won't be the fatty-pants driving up to the nearest fast food joint wasting your money and feeding your family unhealthy and empty junk food. Hey things happen, and you may have a day here and there where things don't actually run smoothly due to your work and family obligations. Knowing this and taking steps to simplify life is a great start. If all plans fail, and from time to time they will, you stop, reevaluate, modify you plans, and possibly compromise. This may lead to...

Chapter 4:

BAD DAYS

Ah, everything is great, then,…..the sh*t hit the fan…There is no way around these! They are going to happen, guaranteed! Kids or no kids, work or no work, one minute everything is great, the next…disaster strikes. Sometimes we just wake up on the wrong side of the bed. It happens! Instead of beating yourself up afterward, the key here is to step back, take a breath, and to think before you act. You can train yourself to do this even on bad days.

Keep in mind that every time you put more crap into your body, the more your body will continue to crave crap. Ho Ho's donuts, ice cream, fried foods, soda = crap! The question is how do you satisfy your cravings and stress without eating the worst crap there is? Now you may think calories are calories. Many nutritionists will argue that calories are calories…hmmm okay, well I can tell you this…if you spike your insulin levels with a boat load of white sugar and empty carbs you can guarantee you will be hungrier than a starved elephant in a desert within a short amount of time. All those empty calories more than likely will also go straight to your fat cells. You know how they say "a moment on the lips a lifetime on the hips?" That has a lot of truth to it. A spike in insulin levels and the rate of digestion highly effects your body composition both directly and indirectly. If you think you will refrain from eating the rest of the day after you scarfed down that box of donuts, I beg to differ with you. Your blood sugar will quickly drop and you will be searching out the next feeding faster than you can get to the nearest donut shop. Also consider that foods laden with garbage such as bleached sugar and preservatives are designed to be addictive. So now not only did you just 'poison' your body with excess processed sugars, you in turn are craving more of the same 'poison'. So yes, calories are a unit of measurement of the energy released by food as we digest it. However, the type of calories you ingest, how slowly they digest, and how you utilize them in the body directly affects your fat cells, insulin, and blood sugar levels in the body. What junk you eat has a direct impact on what you may ingest the rest of the day. And, keep in mind junk has way more calories than healthy food. Try eating a thousand calories of carrots, see how that goes for you. Then see if you can down a thousand calories worth of pizza. I would guess with great confidence the pizza goal would be more easily met! Understanding how junk food and preservatives affect your body is the key to understanding why we need to replace crap food with healthier foods. Of course, you can over eat *any type* of food and still gain weight. Any junk food can leave you with a "junk food hangover" (we affectionately call "gut rot") in which case the next day you feel hungry, tired, constipated, bloated, and crabby. The healthier you normally eat, the worse you feel when you eat junk food. It's a feeling I don't wish on anyone. So what's the alternative? What can one eat to satisfy cravings without ingesting thousands of useless calories and blowing up like a beached whale? Well I will share that secret with you.

What can one eat when a craving strikes and be satisfied WITHOUT ingesting thousands of calories, preservatives, and bleached sugar and flour?

Follow these Simple guidelines:

#1. Keep the junk food out of your house. I bet that's not the first time you have heard that so now you know that is the number one thing to do. If you have to leave to go get your junk fix, you will think twice than if it were sitting in front of your face. Don't play that "I'm buying it for the kids" crap either. The kids shouldn't be eating that crap anyway. Buy them organic yogurt, fruit, applesauce, organic whole wheat pretzels, and healthy organic cereals. We have too many obese children already so do the world a favor and don't let yours get that way. We never had much junk food in my house growing up. We were lucky every few weeks to get a box of cereal that was semi-naughty with some damn colored marshmallows we picked out to eat. Until I went to college, I had never had box mac and cheese or those cardboard noodles that come in a package. So if you never introduce your children to that trash, they will never ask for it.

#2. Realize you are not perfect AND realize it's OK now and then to have some "healthy crap". If you do this, when real junk is placed in front of you, you will eat very little knowing you will feel like a beached whale after your binge. Having a treat or two now and then of organic dark chocolate or homemade gluten free pizza is truly satisfying. Fried junk, and frosting laden cake and sugar drenched ice cream will start to make you sick just thinking about it. It will also taste so rich that you will only be able to eat a small amount. This is the key to your success right here. Get used to the feeling of good food so that the true garbage is unappealing.

#3. Buy organic items whenever you can which includes sweets. Not ideal, but better! Natural sugars don't have the *exact negative effect* on your body as bleached white or brown sugar. Anything made with raw cane sugar or stevia minus the preservatives, dyes, and chemicals is going to have a more positive effect on your body in the long run. Yes, they are still sugar, and if you eat too much you still will feel and get fat! So think again... moderation! Your goal is to forever dump the processed garbage that turns you into something worse that a cocaine addict. And yes that's actually true, I have read studies that have actually proven sugar is more addictive than cocaine (at least to lab rats). Now that you have some healthier versions to choose from, you will feel full longer and know that your digestive system will thank you later.

Sometimes getting creative is all it takes to kill the cravings. Think a bar of dark chocolate with sea salt, coconut yogurt with natural peanut butter, a tablespoon of unsweetened cocoa, and a packet of stevia. Or try some organic coconut milk, the full fat kind, whipped with 2 tablespoons of real maple syrup and fresh strawberries, organic blue corn chips with salsa, gluten free fig bars, or any other moderate serving of organic and/or gluten free treats. You can make gluten free pizza dough and top it with tons of veggies and organic or vegan cheese. Almond, soy, or coconut milk frozen yogurts and treats are also delicious. All of these options are so yummy and have a much better effect on your entire body than fast food or chemical laden junk lining almost every isle of the grocery store. If you ever browse around the organic section of the grocery store, look at what's available and read the labels. See what might work as far as how much you can eat in comparison to the calories ingested.

Here again, just because it's gluten free don't get the impression that it's ok to scarf down a couple boxes of cookies and things will be fine. I'm telling you right now they won't be fine, and you will have the bigger ass to prove it. Our biggest issue with wheat these days is that it is not the wheat that was grown fify years ago. Nothing food wise is what it was fify years ago, however wheat seems to be the target of digestive issues that many authors have written about. You have to decide what is best for you. Some individuals cannot digest or tolerate wheat or dairy while others can. My advice is to experiment by eliminating wheat and/or dairy for a period of a month. Then slowly integrate them back in one at a time to see how you feel. If you feel like crap, then you know to stay away from these common allergens. If you feel fine ingesting one or both of these nutrients, my suggestion is to purchase only organic non-GMO wheat and dairy products and still consume them in moderation. Don't jump on the gluten free "bandwagon" just because your buddy lost 20 lbs. doing so.

Do you remember the "fat free" craze of the 90's? Everyone and their mother were downing bags of gummy type candy thinking "oh these are fat free, it says so!" Yeah and everyone's ass grew three sizes. They may have been "Fat Free" like so many foods are listed even today. But did they check how much sugar was in those "Fat Free" foods? Sugar and extra calories will most definitely diminish your success and add to your waistline even if it is fat free. So just remember, even healthier naughty treats can catch up to you if over eaten just as the other bad crap would. The difference is the organic versions will lack the "pollutants" that you would find in the "other" junk food we normally turn to.

#4. DO NOT go hungry....ever! Plan, plan, plan! Make sure you have eaten before making that shopping trip to the grocery store. I know you have heard that one before but let me beat it into you again, in a good way of course! If you go hungry it's almost a guarantee you will buy some, if not a lot of junk food. As we have discussed, the key is never keep junk in your house even if you think it is "good" junk food. Go out to get it, and before you leave have a smoothie or a tablespoon of nut butter to ease the hunger cravings. Then decide if you "need" your fix. If you follow this, you will see that you won't need to go scarfing down a package of half-moons before you hit home. Use common sense, stop, take a breath, drink some water, have a healthy snack then head out.

#5. Bring snacks for trips and outing. Don't go shopping or golfing with your friends and have nothing to eat with you. Chances are your buddies are going to want to stop and have a bite to eat and possibly a drink. If you have a quality protein bar or small bag of almonds to munch on, you will less likely choose the garbage at the restaurant. If you aren't starving you will pass up the white bread and wait patiently for your veggie soup, salad, or lean meat/fish/poultry with veggies on the side. The best part of this is that you may positively influence them to stop eating like crap and start giving a damn about what they are putting in their bodies. Seeing you glowing and slimming down will drive that point home, and as a group you may decide to support one another in your endeavors.

#6. Axing the Negative Sh*t...Again! Just to drive that point home again, yes, we have been here before.. It is vital that you don't sabotage yourself with negative thoughts. Don't beat yourself up if you have a moment of weakness, it will be ok as long as you focus on your long-term goals! You might feel bloated and fat. You may not want to wear your best clothes and put on a smile. If you have read any other information on the topic of positive thinking, many say "fake it till you make it". And as an avid believer of this, put on your very best and project positivity as someone else always has it much worse than you do.

Food Quantity vs. Calorie Burn

I am just going to put this out there right away... Do not eat all the calories back that you just burned off exercising. You need to be in a caloric deficit to lose fat. You can't play that I can eat everything as long as it's protein or fat bullsh*t. To lose one pound, you need to burn 3,500 calories that is a known fact and you can look it up almost anywhere. Burning off this many calories is almost impossible to do with either workout or diet alone. It is recommended that one does not go too far into a calorie deficit for too long of a period or the body will assume "starvation mode". If your body thinks its starving a couple of things will happen. Number one, you will store fat because your body will fight to insulate itself when it thinks no nutrients are coming its way. Number two, your body will start breaking down that protein in your muscle tissue to feed itself. Less muscle equals slower metabolism. Get the point? To prevent the above from occurring, keep in mind is that the food you choose to eat and the quantities determines about 80% of your success while busting your butt at the gym only produces 20% results. Because you cannot create a serious calorie deficit without mega overtraining and potentially injuring yourself (not to mention you are seriously raising your levels of cortisol; the stress hormone), you must monitor your intake of chow. You could literally work out for five hours per day and if you are stuffing your face, you most definitely won't be losing any fat. Does this mean you should count calories or write in a food journal? If that is something you need to do then the answer is yes. For some people, that is the best way to monitor their intake and be accountable for it. I have never counted calories, but have used a food journal. Writing down what I ate all the time became stressful in and of itself, however, doing it for a few days allowed me to see some general patterns that I needed to address. Some people use apps on their smartphone to track both food and exercise. The most effective way to track food intake I have discovered is to portion things correctly, know what you eating for the next day, and have a good handle on the calorie content and nutritional value of foods. As you become more education on the calories and nutritional content, you also become more savvy in selecting high volume lower calorie foods (i.e.: fruits and vegetables, lean proteins) naturally. It becomes like brushing your teeth. This sounds pretty general in regards to calorie control; however, I have had my body fat to mere 8% without journaling or counting calories. I didn't weigh or measure my food. I simply educated myself on what to eat and when so that the bulk of my food intake was earlier in the day and immediately after working out. My starchy carbohydrate intake was ingested early in the day and immediately after a workout. I still enjoy starchy carbs such as sweet potatoes as they offered volume and satiety for fewer calories instead of ingesting one cup of processed pasta that would leave me hungry in hour. To this day I still utilize such practices and incorporate lean animal proteins, nut butters and oils, ghee, fruits, veggies, nut milks, and use whey and plant based protein shakes to "measure" my intake via portion control.

Look at some of those people in the gym that we discussed earlier. No you shouldn't be nasty and judgmental. But take a look and realize you want something different for yourself. People that work out every day should see results! Results for some people who are already fit and lean could be maintenance. For others it may mean losing moderate to serious fat while gaining lean muscle mass. If this is not happening, something is wrong. The same workout at the same intensity day in day out, and overfeeding leads to zero results. And don't start going crazy on me and think you are going to start marathon training just to lose body fat. If you really want to run a marathon or participate in a triathlon, more power to you. However, over exercising can have just as much as a negative effect as under exercising. Trust me on this. Your body will quickly adapt to the amount of exercise you are doing, and through this adaptation at the cellular level, you won't be burning as many calories anymore, not to mention you will be highly over trained unless you already are engaging in this type of rigorous regimen. So if you have the innate desire to train for such a competition, you will have to monitor your energy levels as well as your food intake to make sure you are eating and training with the idea that you will more than likely lose a little or maintain your weight during the course of your training... Training for specific events is a whole other story. Whether you are body building or running a marathon each event has a specific training and eating protocol. It is best not to approach training for any performance event without researching how to eat and train to maximize performance and minimize injury to the body. I can tell you this, MOST sports do not require an excess of body fat in order to perform well. Contrary to popular thought, this also applies to power lifting events. Fat does not move the weight, muscles do. Having a little more fat for cushion is fine, but carrying around 30 pounds of excess fat and benching or squatting your max weight is dangerous to your blood pressure, joints, etc. So work at keeping yourself in a healthy lower body fat category. This not only improves your aesthetics but also improves your performance in almost any sport or athletic event.

Getting back to eating again, another good rule of thumb so to speak is to enjoy one meal a week that is "bad". This can mean you splurge at a wedding or other event such as a barbeque or birthday. After all, you should have a little bit of fun. One "fun" meal a week will not only keep you sane but give you something to look forward to. Oddly enough, overeating once in a while will actually speed up your metabolism for a period of time. This idea goes back to that starvations mode concept. It is better not to be in a large calorie deficit for more than 7 days. So here is your freebie meal day...not the whole day..just one meal! Without getting all chemistry on you, there are a variety of chemical reactions taking place that will create this increased metabolic effect in the body. To save you the boring scientific details of such reactions, we will just refer to this phenomenon as a change in your levels of leptin. Leptin is another hormone within your body that drops when you are reducing your caloric intake. This slight overfeeding technique will not work if you are taking too many leftovers home and scarfing down crap regularly. So keep that in check and keep it to once a week and only once a week. If you do happen to screw it up, which we all do from time to time, I will tell you again, don't beat yourself up. No, it's not okay to be an avid garbage can, but giving up is not the answer. Everything you think and do counts as a learning experience. So essentially, you need to quit your bitching and crying and move on. If you stand there whining about how you will be eternally overweight, guess what will happen to you? You will never lose anything, or worse, you will lose and put on weight like a yo-yo. On the flip side, if you chose to believe you can achieve whatever you wish and put your thoughts into, sky is the limit. Get back to your normal routine, don't punish yourself, but don't let yourself fall into being a slacker. It's not ok to be mediocre. Don't buy into the poisonous thinking that many people live by thinking fat is beautiful and everyone should get a trophy. NONSENSE! It is not healthy for your heart, joints, liver, pancreas, colon etc. to be fat, and you have to work hard and bust you're a$$ for that trophy no one should be handing it to you! Positivity and hard work make your accomplishments worthwhile; not getting everything handed to you on a silver platter. Re-read and remember this for those times you are thinking of quitting.

Chapter 5:

Who Says Vitamins and Supplements are bad for you?

Now, I am not asking you to use your body for science here and test out every supplement on the market with no rhyme or reason. However, if you take away absolutely nothing else from this book, please just consider this... The "powers that be" out there will always look to keep you uninformed, fat, medicated, and addicted to garbage food that rots your insides. Many vitamins and supplements that actually "work" are often thwarted and found to be unsafe, not to mention ridiculed and then suddenly taken off the market. Go back to our discussion on tobacco products. It's amazing what sh*t people will put in their mouth to get their "fix", yet they are afraid of a damn vitamin. "Cancer sticks" are available for sale to individuals age 18 and over relentlessly causing oral as well as lung cancer. What's worse, if you are near the a$$ who is smoking one, you are at risk as well! If you ever really think about it, it's amazing that a product that has absolutely no health benefits and can kill you and others around you is still allowed to be sold, yet we bag on vitamins and supplements because one or two goofballs used their body as a laboratory. So with great disregard, just keep in mind "those people" who have interests that have nothing to do with your health are supportive and promote the selling of well-known cancerous substances. This as we have discussed satisfies that almighty cash flow into their pockets. Without spending too much time discussing the disgusting methods the "higher-ups" not only promote but endorse, let's just take it for face value that no one is going to invest in your health and wellbeing like you can so get informed. How you will do that is however going to be tricky. Many so-called "health" magazines and online resources are heavily controlled by "those people"... and you know who they are. I am going to throw my mother under the bus for a minute here as she is a classic violator of this phenomenon. She will inform me of the latest and greatest as far as weight loss or other health related topics spewing countless useless facts regarding how high fructose corn syrup has been "proven" to be safe for human consumption. Sure it has! If I wanted to poison you do you think I would be spouting off negative facts about what you were to ingest? I think not! Of course all of the fake sugar, high fructose corn syrup, and medications are safe! Research has proven it! Blah blah blah...research is flawed, research can be altered or even lied about to keep products on the shelves and keep you and me addicted to them. Don't believe me? Re-read the sections on the cigarettes... Now you know. Many individuals who are aware of all of the crap that is fed to us have attempted to put it out there so people know what they are truly up against in regards to their health. Many times the publication is confiscated or bashed publicly to the point that the individual appears to be a "quack" or "witch doctor". Keep in mind choosing the road less traveled sometimes raises a few eyebrows. People may think you are a nut case for getting a colonic and tell you that it's horrible for you and that you are going to rip your colon. Just realize that type of ignorance is just that, ignorance. We can only live and hope that people come around and realized their bodies are not garbage disposals. As far as educating yourself, there are many other publications even more extensive than this that can help you on your way. My suggestion first is to find a well-trained holistic and/or naturopathic doctor in your area. Depending on your location, they may be difficult to find. I do know that many of them practice online, in which case you could consult with him or her regarding specific issues you are experiencing and they may provide you with a viable solution. Unfortunately, medical insurance doesn't cover these options, however in the long run; saving your pennies for the more appropriate treatment is priceless. In some cases, there are conventional medical doctors who have adopted the holistic approach knowing their patients are more educated about their health; they don't prescribe medications as often as others. Yet, it may be difficult to find a practitioner who will prescribe essential oils or vitamin therapy for your ailments. You may also consider soliciting the expertise of an acupuncturist or holistic nutritionists who may advise you to utilize certain supplements or food as therapy.

As far as solving the supplement mystery, you could pull your hair out trying to figure out what to safely ingest. We have already discussed that taking a whole green foods vitamin and essential fatty acids is never a bad thing. You may have been led to believe if you are eating a well-balanced diet that's enough, however, we now know that even with organic food; the environment just isn't allowing us to reap all the benefits of our food. The air we breathe, the soil, job environment, even our homes can cause our bodies to work overtime processing all those free radicals. Keep in mind vitamins do not replace your food intake, they simply supplement it ensuring you are getting everything you need to function optimally. Just as I have said before, some people think "oh this is useless, I am buying and taking vitamins and just excrete what I don't use". Yes, you will excrete what you don't use as food as well. That's completely normal. In my opinion, I would rather eliminate what I don't use vitamin wise rather than discover I'm deficient in one or more of them. Especially those related to bone health.

One of my favorite green food vitamins also contains probiotics. This is a great option for those of us who are not into swallowing twenty pills a day or are on a budget. Probiotics and digestive enzymes when taken together are excellent for intestinal health and the proper breakdown and absorption of food.

As we age, we tend to lose some of our digestive enzymes, our stomach acids can decrease, and we can even experience issues with absorption, excretion, develop food or other allergies, and possibly have bacteria, parasites, or issues such as leaky gut syndrome. Probiotics and digestive enzymes are great resources for addressing these issues. Again, getting the specifics on what your body really needs at the point you are at in your life can really take some of the guess work out of what you should be taking. That's why I continue to stress the importance of a holistic nutritionist who can find and address your needs. Search out a nutritionist who uses biofeedback or some other modality to analyze your personal needs. The nutritionist I work with uses a biofeedback machine to analyze the body and determine deficiencies. It may be eating for your blood type that works, lowering your intake of gluten, dairy, or starchy carbs, or working on eating more green vegetables. There is also a way to test your DNA via swabbing the inside of your cheek to find out what types of food agree with your system and those that don't.

The Other Side of the Coin

Now, let's not get confused here, if you are experiencing a heart condition, or have incurred an infection, or have a true medical emergency, do not hesitate to utilize conventional medicine. Unfortunately, all the essential oils and vitamins in the world are not going to stop a heart attack in its tracks. Certain life practices may PREVENT having such an unfortunate condition, but we can't argue with getting yourself to a medical doctor in an emergency. There are many cases in which you NEED to see a medical doctor and be treated with actual medication. You may even have to have surgery. Don't get me wrong, I completely am all for conventional medicine, medication, and surgery WHEN NEEDED. That's the problem, if it were only used when it was absolutely necessary, this whole publication wouldn't really need to exist. We do need medical doctors for everything from stitches to staph infections, repairing ligaments and tendons, removing tumors, organ transplants, etc. These modern medical procedures are all miracles and have contributed to our longevity. What burns my behind (and yours as well) is when useless and harmful medications are prescribed to either perfectly healthy people, or those who are actually in dire need of an exercise program, physical therapy, chiropractic, or a huge diet change. People are conned into believing that pain medication or the like actually "cures" their condition. So many individuals are prescribed crap to deal with their crap, which of course...equals more crap! Another very important fact to keep in mind is that most medical doctors have very little training and experience in nutrition and exercise. Unless they actually have educated themselves or are highly active and nutritionally conscious, you are not going to get much from an MD on how to live a healthy lifestyle. They predominantly practice diagnosis and prescribing tests to determine your condition and consequently a medication is prescribed. I have never seen a doctor write a prescription for 3 days a week of 1 hour of physical exercise, though I'd be pretty impressed to see doctors adopting such practices. Ideally, this would be the case that modern medicine worked synergistically with holistic therapy, nutrition and exercise. However, if it did, a lot of agencies would be put out of business. So it's up to you and me to become educated, resourceful, mindful, and know what our health options really are.

To exacerbate this issue, I was once told by an overweight doctor to "make sure I was living a healthy lifestyle". After giving her a strange look, I realized I was speechless. I couldn't even form the words "are you kidding me" to express my disbelief of what I just heard. This is one of the top ten reasons I have chosen to write this book. This is why I want you to be educated. Even if you think I am a complete moron and have no business writing this publication, if you can do one simple thing for yourself it should be to learn about your body. Learn how it functions, from hormones to blood sugar levels. Know what your blood pressure should be, understand how blood cholesterol functions, what LDL's versus HDL's. Take responsibility for your own health and body and never let anyone take that away from you. Ask questions before accepting prescriptions, and above all, seek out safer, natural alternatives.

The Uphill Battle: Your Body's Reaction to Your Efforts

Ok, now let's get down to the real dirty stuff. Despite all your honest efforts, there will be times when your body doesn't respond exactly the way you want it to. Here is a random example of what I am talking about. You start ingesting more fiber in an effort to keep your colon and cholesterol in check; you hear it's a good idea. Great! Then, you realize a few days later you are so bloated your stomach looks like a beach ball, you are retaining a gallon of water, and you haven't pooped in days. The worst part of this above and beyond how you feel is the emotional turmoil that begins happening within you. Your spirit is shot, your will power down the drain, and that half gallon of ice cream looks and feels like your only hope for happiness. However, after your compulsive binge you are back to square one feeling like a beached whale, and in no way adding to the health and well-being of your body. So stop right there, put down the spoon, and listen up. There are a couple things here that you need to keep in mind before you go off on the deep end..

#1: Remember, your body is not always going to function **PERFECTLY**. If you think just because you are changing things that a magical fairy will come down and immediately "fix" you, good luck, let me know when you find her and send her my way. Making changes will wreak havoc on the status quo of your body and cause you to experience a few changes that are less desirable at first. Even when you do everything right, you may still have a transition period where your body is "holding" some water, fat, etc. Remember exercising causes micro-tears in the muscles which leads to some swelling and stiffness. Exercise also can cause lactic acid build-up in the muscles which will also need to be processed by the liver. Waste products and the release of toxins from everywhere will sometimes make you sick; give you sinus issues, headaches, constipation, foul smelling urine, night sweats, sleeplessness, or a cold or flu. Sounds like one of those pharmaceutical commercials doesn't it! Don't freak out, this will pass. Much of what you are experiencing is just a "side effect" of your body releasing toxins. The good news is that unlike the medications, you will actually begin to benefit greatly from all your efforts for the rest of your life!

#2. Don't change too many things at once, AND don't overdo it! There are a couple of reasons for this. Number one is the above. If you change too much at once, you many find yourself sick and miserable depending on how toxic your body is and how much of those toxins are now being released into your blood stream. Second, if you change too much at once it's difficult to determine exactly what is working and not working. A classic example of this is working out. Everyone wants to change so much at once especially in regards to adding time to their workout that not only do they end up injured potentially, but they also have to keep adding more time to their workouts to get the same effect. All of this is not necessary. You have four weapons in regards to exercise. Frequency, intensity, time, and type. The best advice I can give you is to change the intensity, then the type, then the frequency, then lastly the time. Don't do 2 hour workouts. You can't possibly maintain an effective intensity that long anyway. Unless you decide to train for a specific event, use the increased time as your last resort. What I mean by all of this is when you notice your body is not changing as much anymore which will usually happen within 4-6 weeks of you starting an exercise regimen, change what you're doing and how intensely you're doing it, not the amount of time you spend. Go through your weight circuit faster, add more weight, do some sprinting and jogging instead of just jogging, add some plyometrics to your workout in between weight sets or jogging or biking. There are plenty of resources online and APPS for your smart phone that will incorporate this variety into your workout.

#3. Accept that everything will take time, hard work, and patience. I would love to tell you all of this will go perfectly smooth, but that is hardly ever the case. And not to go off on a tangent, but we all need to be patient and respectful of our bodies and its timelines for adjusting. For women, we must remember our bodies function differently than men. Menstruation, menopause, all the crazy hormonal changes that go on in our bodies can have a negative effect from time to time on our efforts. As for men, as testosterone levels decrease, muscle mass decreases, and therefore for both men and women, it is essential to keep the muscle mass on and keep body fat levels low. You will feel better, the fog will subside, and your eyes will begin to shine, so do some deep breathing and meditation and keep your positivity on the rise.

#4. The life long journey lesson. Here we go again. For the rest of your beautiful life, you will have cravings, you will screw up once in a while, you may even quit, back track, or feel all your efforts are worthless. But trust me, the days you are most lethargic, you are craving the salt, sugar, or alcohol, those are the times to take a step back, distract yourself, meditate, journal, call a friend, walk your dog, or if you can get a massage or use a sauna. Walk away and try treating yourself in different ways so that the reward or "go to" item when you are feeling overwhelmed is NOT food. You can retrain your body and mind to dump the crap for good. The less you eat sugar, the less you crave it. The same goes for other substances such as alcohol, salt, and excessive carbohydrates.

You Can't Afford to be "Poo-pooing" It

When I have personally trained people at the gym, I enjoyed using humor and a touch of sarcasm to motivate and inspire them. I am not one for yelling in someone's face and threatening them into submission or guilting them into working harder on their bodies. However, in each client I have worked with, I had to be a real and honest person with them letting them know repeating the same old routine in any area of their life expecting different results is the definition of insanity. So I will continue to say this time and time again. You can't be a slacker in your own mind body and soul. You will say ugh! But I just want to relax and not think about this stuff all the time, I'm becoming obsessed! I don't want you to have to think about it all the time, in fact, I want it to be so automatic you don't have to think at all. At first, you have to put the time in. It may feel like a job. To me, this part of my life if automatic, I eat and exercise like I brush my teeth. It wasn't always like this, but it is not an inherent part of my existence. We all struggle with something. To share a more personal experience, I struggle with meditation. I have vowed to be more in touch with my higher self as I know it brings me peace and a connection that I deeply wish to have with the universe. I have very little patience yet have a sincere desire to be connected to my soul. I still meditate every day twice a day. I listen to a guided meditation, I focus, and I yearn deeply for that spiritual connection. Therefore, I don't and won't give up. Deep within me I have profoundly

68

committed to being connected to my higher self, and that deep commitment is something all of us can chose in any area of our lives. Committing to yourself is always the first step in your journey. Once you have committed to what it is that you truly want without "poo-pooing" around it you will start to see amazing things happening in your life. You simply can't waste your life sitting on the couch watching reality TV or playing games on your phone and expect to have time to work out, chill out, eat properly, and take care of your home and family. Learn to disconnect from what is not necessary to your well-being, find your higher self, and learn to engage in activities that are more suitable to enriching your life. Spend time in nature hiking, walking, biking, swimming, camping, kayaking, paddle boarding, rollerblading, disc golf, mini golf, regular golf! If you experience snowy winters, take up snowshoeing, cross country skiing, downhill skiing or snowboarding, or winter hiking. Get out with your family and spend some quality time engaging instead of existing. Regardless of your level of income or athletic prowess, most of these activities are inexpensive and just require you to round up your loved ones. Taking a walk and enjoying nature is cheap yet priceless to your well-being and social interaction with your family. If you don't have family around you, go enjoy the peace of a forest, jog or walk through it, climb a mountain, breathe in the fresh, crisp air in the morning, or if you are super ambitious, train for an event! A friend of mine and I trained for a ten mile hill race by taking her son in the jogging stroller out in her neighborhood that was filled with steep hills. Each of us took turns pushing the jogging stroller up those crazy hills! Hey you have to do what you have to do. We started our runs at 6 am sharp or if that didn't work, we ran after school. Either way, we got it done and ran that grueling ten mile race side by side earning a medal for completing it in under an hour and a half. As you can see, anything is possible. Don't underestimate yourself and settle for "I can't" or "I don't have time". Let's face it, if you don't do it now when will you? Kick yourself in the pants, make goals, start, keep going, and never give up.

RE-Cap and RE-Lease

Now that you have read the above information that I have had the pleasure of sharing with you, it is your job to get out there and get started. Regardless of how large or small of a change you make right now today, any change for the better will indefinitely lead you to a more fulfilling healthy life. At this point, I think you get the point that sitting on you're a$$ will only cause it to get larger while your insides continue to rot creating unholy hell on your existence. I want you to feel better, look better, and function better. In conjunction with that, I also want to provide you with the cold hard no bullsh*t truth about what is needed and necessary for you to finally drop the excuses and be successful from here on out. Someone once shared with me that success in any area of your life is 90% mind set, and 10% the work you put into it. That goes for your health, the success of an athletic endeavor, a business, etc. Put plainly, this sh*t ain't easy. So begin by releasing your self-doubts and get you're a$$ out there and start living your life. You will notice lots of changes when you consciously make that decision. Say right now to yourself "I consciously choose to live a healthier, happier, more productive existence". Write it down, repeat it, and never lose site or where you are going with that notion. Start by utilizing what you have learned in the book right this minute. I can tell you I have learned so much from networking in my own town. When you find one holistic person such as a Reiki Master or nutritionist, they will know others who can help spur you down many different avenues. As a result, you may discover a great acupuncturist, massage therapist, or chiropractor. You may discover a great place to purchase vitamins and organic foods. Local organizations such as yoga studios, wellness centers, spas, etc., have workshops, classes, and programs that you can partake in to educate yourself and get in touch with like- minded people. The fun part is that you continue to meet so many neat people you begin to make friends within that circle of individuals.

I hope you have enjoyed the information and the manner in which I have shared it with you. I am generally a no-nonsense, drama free person, who speaks in language that even I can understand! I am not an English major, and this book is not professionally edited so that I sound "smarter" but in fact I published it myself to allow my sincere personality and passions shine through. I can only hope that you come to feel as passionate and interested in your well-being as I am. I once again sincerely thank each and every person who reads this book, and hope that if you do have any further questions that you contact me for more information. Now get your body and mind REWIRED....

The Best of Health on Your Life's Journey!!!

Sources and Resources

Acupuncture

www.acupuncture.com

www.acupuncture-points.org

Adrenal Fatigue

www.adrenalfatigue.org

Nutrition and Wellness Books

8 Weeks to Optimum Health: *A Proven Program for Taking Full Advantage of Your Body's Natural Healing Power.* 2007. Dr. Andrew Weil. Publisher. Ballantine Books. 320 pgs. ISBN-10# 034549802X. ISBN-13 # 978-0345498021.

Juice Fasting and Detoxification. *Using the Healing Power of Fresh Juice to Feel Young and Look Great.* By Steve Meyerowitz. 2002. 154 pgs. ISBN# 1-878736-65-5

The Detox Diet. By Elson M Haas, MD. 1996. 128 pgs. ISBN# 0890878145.

Guide to Eating Gluten Free. By The Mayo Clinic. 2014. 111 pgs. Published by Time Home Entertainment Inc. 1271 Avenue of the Americas, New York, NY 10020

The Blood Sugar Solution. *Activate Your Body's Natural Ability to Burn Fat and Lose Weight Fast.* 2014. By Mark Hyman, MD. Published by Little Brown and Company. 352 pgs. ISBN-10 # 0316230022. ISBN-13 # 978-0316230025

Chiropractic Wellness

www.yourspine.com/Chiropractic/Health+Benefits+Of+Chiropractic+Adjustments+Affect+Entire+Body.aspx

www.thejoint.com/health-benefits

Colon Hydrotherapy

www.colonhealth.net

www.coloncleanse.net

Exercise Resources

www.hiittraining .net

www.intervaltraining.net/HiitTraining-30.html

www.livestrong.com

www.spartan.com

www.crossfit.com

Food, Gadgets, and Local Farms

The Thug Kitchen Cookbook. 2014. Rodale Books. 240 pgs. www.thugkitchen.com. ISBN-10 #1623363586, ISBN-13 #13-978-1623363581

www.localharvest.org

www.rawtimes.com

www.vitamix.com

www.ninjakitchen.com

www.spartan.com

Healing Resources/Holistic Health

American Holistic Health Association. P.O. Box 17400, Anaheim, CA 92817-7400. 714-779-6152. www.ahha.org. Resource for holistic practitioners.

www.naturalcures.com

www.drweil.com

www.chetday.com

Infrared Sauna Therapy Information

http://www.globalhealingcenter.com/natural-health/health-benefits-of-far-infrared-therapy/

www.sunlighten.com

Inspiration and Motivation

www.mindmovies.com

Change Your Thoughts, Change Your Life. 2009. Dr. Wayne Dyer. Publisher. Hay House. Pgs. 416. ISBN-10 # 140191750X. ISBN-13 # 978-1401917500

My Philosophy on Successful Living. 2012. Jim Rohn. Publisher. No Dream Too Big LLC. 64 pgs.

ISBN-10 #0983841594. ISBN-13 # 978-0983841593

Never In Your Wildest Dreams. 2013 by Natalie Ledwell. Sherpa Press Publishing. 193 pgs.

ASIN-B00C6NHO01

The Law of Attraction. 2006. Esther and Jerry Hicks. Publisher. Hay House. 224 pgs. ISBN-10 # 1401912273. ISBN-13 # 978-1401912277.

Wished Fulfilled: *Mastering the Art of Manifesting.* 2012. Dr. Wayne Dyer. Publisher. Hay House. 203 pgs. ISBN-10 # 9781401937270. ISBN-13 # 978-1401937270.

You Can Heal Your Life. 1984. Louise Hay. Publisher. Hay House. 272 pgs. www.lousisehay.com. www.healyourlife.com. ISBN-10 #9780937611012. ISBN-13 # 978-0937611012

Healing Spas and Resorts

New Age Health Spa. Neversink, NY 12765. 845-985-7601. www.NewAgeHealthspa.com

Red Mountain Resort. Ivin, Utah 84738. 877-246-4453. www.redmountainresort.com

Leptin

www.yourhormones.info/hormones/leptin.aspx

Massage Therapy

www.massagetherapy.com/articles/index.php?article_id=468

www.mayoclinic.org/healthy-living/stress-management/in-depth/massage/art-20045743

Nutritionist (holistic)

Patricia Serrao, LLC. P.O. Box 121. Liverpool, NY 13088. 315-461-9961

Reiki

www.reiki.org/faq/WhatIsReiki.html
www.reiki-for-holistic-health.com/

Social Networking

www.meetup.com

Vitamins/Supplements/Natural Foods

Vitamin Warehouse, www.vitaglo.com, 3990 New Court Ave, Syracuse, NY 13206, 315-437-4542

Renew Life. Clearwater FL 33765. 800-830-4778. 813-871-3200. www.renewlife.com

Green Foods Corporation. www.greenfoods.com

www.ingramcontent.com/pod-product-compliance
Lightning Source LLC
Chambersburg PA
CBHW070605290526
45790CB00002B/795